Make Dementia Your B*tch!

An Easy Guide to Understanding and Handling Dementia-Driven Behaviors

Rita Jablonski, PhD, CRNP, FAAN, FGSA

DementiaCentric Solutions LLC
Rita Jablonski, PhD, CRNP, FAAN, FGSA
1401 Doug Baker Blvd
STE 107-185
Birmingham, AL 35242

dementiacentric@gmail.com
www.dementiacetricsolutions.com

Make Dementia Your B*tch! / Rita Jablonski. —1st ed.
Paperback ISBN: 979-8-9852744-0-0
eBook ISBN: 979-8-9852744-1-7

Contents

Don't Skip!

I'm sorry you are going through this dementia journey. Please understand that I am not here to minimize or make fun of a devastating disease, despite the edgy and profane title of my book. Dementia is a nasty bitch of a disease, and I want to help you THRIVE as a caregiver. Let's face it—your loved one's quality of life depends on your quality of life. If you are equipped to understand and handle behaviors, your caregiving path will be smoother. If your caregiving path is smoother and more pleasant, your loved one's dementia journey will be positive despite the challenges.

The goal of MDYB is to help family caregivers of people living with dementia to understand the "why" behind the behaviors while supplying the "how" for handling the behaviors. Examples of these behaviors faced by family caregivers include repetition (also known as Same Damn Question), refusals, mixed-up memories (sometimes called "confabulation" in the scientific literature), anxiety, agitation, anger, wandering, shadowing, and assertions that "I'm fine, there is nothing wrong with my memory," which is known as anosognosia (more on that later) in the clinical arena.

The content in this book comes from 40 years of providing nursing care to adults with dementia; 20 years as a funded researcher, testing different approaches to dementia care; almost 10 years as a nurse practitioner in a Memory Clinic; and personal experience as a family caregiver. Please note that the examples and anecdotes in this book do not come from any one clinical or research encounter. If you recognize yourself or your family member in any of this content, it is because I have done my job and am tackling the common problems experienced by family caregivers. No matter how unusual or bizarre a situation may seem to you or even another clinician, I've seen at least a dozen situations equally (or more so) unusual or bizarre in my travels. When names are used for persons with dementia or their caregivers, the names are made up—pseudonyms.

There are two things I hate about many caregiver books that I've tried to fix in this book. The first one is that many caregiving books describe behaviors, but never provide anything useful about how to prevent or manage these behaviors. There is a shit-ton of strategies in this book! The second thing is the use of dry, boring, technical language. Yes, I will use the correct terms but I will explain them. What I really want is for this book to feel like a conversation. If any of the family caregivers with whom I work read this book, they should feel like they are sitting in one of my exam rooms or am on the phone with me. I also believe in humor and authenticity. Humor is a beautiful thing and laughter really does improve brain chemistry. If you find my language or humor offensive, stop here and go read the boring stuff.

…which leads me to my word choices:

- *Dementia.* I use "dementia" because it is a catch-all word for the many different types of dementias. I will introduce you to them in the first chapter.

- *Caregiver.* "Caregiver" is the common word used both in the lay and scientific literature to describe the individual helping the person with dementia. Some prefer "caregiver" or "care manager." Despite the debate, I will remain old school and use "caregiver."

- *Behaviors.* In the hallowed halls of academia, where people have a lot of time on their hands to argue over words and punctuation, there is a current raging debate about how to label dementia-related behaviors. "Behavioral and psychological symptoms of dementia" and "care-resistant behavior" is considered by some to be "insulting" to the person living with dementia. The family caregivers with whom I work couldn't give a rat's rump what the behaviors are called, they just want the behaviors to STOP and desire the tools to prevent and reduce said behaviors. Again, I'm ignoring the debate and sticking with words that make sense to you, the reader.

- *Family.* In this book, "family" refers to families of blood, bondage (marriage), or belief (chosen family). Many of us have friends who would give us one of their kidneys and siblings who do not even know or care if we are alive, much less if we need a kidney. This may be particularly true for my LGBTQ readers who face some completely unique caregiving challenges

Some of the strategies described in this book are on my YouTube channel, also called "Make Dementia Your Bitch" (http://https://www.youtube.com/channel/UCo0fo1nY6TDI8I-8Bp8zAyQ). You may also want to listen to my podcast, which is found on 10 different platforms including Spotify, Audible, Apple Music, Google Play, Castbox, and a bunch of others. I offer free webinars throughout the year. All of my free stuff is housed on the Make Dementia Your B*tch website (http://makedementiayourbitch.com). Stop by and sign up for weekly newsletters; this way, you will always be the first to know when something new and awesome is coming!

Learning all of this information may be very overwhelming. I periodically offer live dementia behavior workshops online. I can help you identify the best strategies for difficult behaviors and help you personalize the strategies so that they make sense for your family member! Dementia behavior coaching or signing up for a dementia behavior course is no different than working with a personal training, taking a yoga class, or hiring someone to teach you how to play a musical instrument! Dementia behavior coaching or a dementia behavior course will save you time, energy, and a lot of aggravation and frustration! Check out the options on my course site, https://dementiacentricsolutions.com. I also work privately with individual clients. You can reach me at info@makedementiayourbitch.com and we can set up a time to talk!

Thank you, caregivers, for the hard work you do. The latest estimates from the Alzheimer's Association place your numbers in the USA around 15 million (I think there are way more) and you are providing billions of dollars in unpaid care. If every one of you got up today and decided, "I'm done," and dropped your loved one off at a hospital or fire station or police station, this country would come to a grinding halt. And some days, when I listen to the latest politico talk about the "opioid epidemic" that only affects 2 million people, I wish everyone would make that gesture to shake these political dudes and dudettes out of their fantasy world. But I know you are out there. I hear you. I see you. I notice you at restaurants, stores, houses of worship, and while walking my dog. Let's go forth and make Dementia YOUR Bitch!

PART 1
DEMENTIA CARE BASICS

CHAPTER 1

Meet the Common Dementias

"Dementia" refers to ANY ongoing, permanent, and worsening memory problem. Alzheimer's dementia, Vascular dementia, dementia with Lewy bodies, and frontotemporal dementia are ALL types of dementia. One way to think about this is to talk about cars. If I ask you, "What kind of car do you drive?", you may respond by saying, "Honda," or "Ford." "Car" refers to any type of gas-powered, multi-person vehicle; Ford or Honda refers to a specific make, or type, of a car. We can even get more specific and discuss models within a specific make. You may not only own a Ford, but you may drive a Ford Fusion, a Ford Explorer, or a Ford Mustang (lucky you!) Some dementias have subtypes, just like makes have models. Frontal-temporal dementia, for example, has 2 common subtypes: behavioral variant and primary progressive aphasia.

All cars have one thing in common: they are powered by an engine that moves the wheels. All the dementias have one thing in common: brain shrinkage (also known as neurodegeneration). What differs between the dementias are the patterns of brain shrinkage and the underlying reasons for the brain (or nerve cell) damage.

Alzheimer's Dementia (AD)

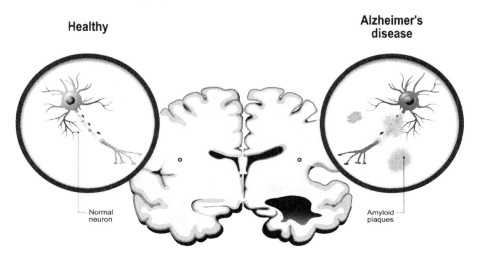

This is the most popular one, probably because it was the first one described a hundred years ago by Dr. Alois Alzheimer. People with AD have progressive (meaning it gets worse over time) memory loss. The memory loss may first involve minor things, like forgetting something that they were just told. As the disease worsens, the person forgets how to do things (called "praxis") in the reverse order in which he or she learned the task. Most of us learned tasks in the following order: swallow, feed ourselves with our fingers, crawl, walk, talk, use utensils to eat, go potty, dress ourselves, brush our teeth, tie our shoes, read, ride a bike, drive, and balance a checkbook. With AD, the tasks are "lost" in the order in which they were learned. I have seen individuals who were fluent in several languages lose their ability to speak and understand those languages, starting with the language learned latest in life. AD can occur early, that is, in individuals under the age of 65 (early onset AD) or later in life (late-onset AD in persons 65 years of age or older). Early onset AD is usually hereditary, and the genes can be identified. Late-onset AD is due to a mix of genetic risk and lifestyle choices. For more information, please visit the Alzheimer's Association's web site http://www.alz.org/ and Alzheimer's of Central Alabama website. http://alzca.org/

Vascular Dementia

Vascular dementia refers to changes in memory and the ability to do things because of stroke-related brain damage. I like to use the image of a highway that gets a lot of traffic. Years of HEAVY traffic can cause a highway to get damaged and develop potholes. Years of high cholesterol and high blood pressure in the blood vessels all over the body, including the brain, can cause damage to those blood vessels. The blood vessels stop sending blood to the parts of the brain, and those parts die off. When the neurons die off, the brain shrinks like the picture above. Members of minority groups who are at higher risk for diabetes and high blood pressure are at higher risk for vascular dementia.

High blood pressure. High blood pressure happens when arteries, the blood vessels that carry oxygenated blood to all body parts including the brain, tighten up or constrict. Cigarette smoking causes blood vessels to become smaller. The smaller the vessel, the longer it takes for blood cells to deliver oxygen and take away waste. Think about it. Would you rather be part of a large group walking through a giant door, or part of a large group of people are trying to get through a small doorway? In the second case, the crowd bunches up and a line forms because people can only move through the small door single-file. If the doorway was double or triple the size, the people could move through it more quickly.

High cholesterol. High levels of cholesterol result in "sludge" along the sides of your blood vessels. The blood cells bump into the sides of the vessels and cause damage. Some get stuck in the sludge can create clots. This damage plus the clots cause blood vessels to close off. If brain cells cannot get oxygen, they die.

Diabetes. Uncontrolled blood sugar "candy-coats" the red blood cells. These cells get a hard shell on them, and they rip into the blood vessels as the cells travel through the body. The body tries to repair the rips in the blood vessels by creating clots. Sometimes, the clots do the trick and absorb, leaving some scar tissue. Sometimes, the clots break off and lodge in smaller downstream blood vessels. The brain cells being fed by the smaller vessel die off.

Brain damage over time. High blood pressure, high cholesterol, and diabetes, if not controlled, create problems with oxygen-rich blood coming to various parts of the body, including the brain. When someone has a stroke, the reason is either a blood vessel blockage (this happens most of the time) or a brain bleed from a burst blood vessel. Depending on the part of the brain that is damaged, and the size of the damage, and you may see memory problems plus problems with making and understanding speech.

Cognitive reserve. Cognitive reserve is the build up of neurons in the brains. Cognitive reserve is like muscle in weight lifters. Let's say I have 2 people standing next to each other. They are both 70 years old. "Arnold" pumped iron, ran marathons, and ate healthy. He has arms and legs that look like massive tree trunks because of all the muscle he built up over 60 years of lifestyle choices. Next to Arnold is another 70-year-old who went to the gym three times a week, kept his weight in the "normal" range, and whose diet was pretty good. "Sheldon" has muscle but nothing like Arnold! Both get sick and are unable to exercise. One year later, we stand the two of them together. Arnold still looks buff. Even though he lost 50% of his muscle, his tree trunk arms and legs are still toned and impressive. On the other hand, Sheldon looks like a twig—like you could break him in half. He also lost 50% of his muscle but he didn't have as much extra muscle as Arnold. You could say that Arnold had more muscular reserve.

People can build up "cognitive reserve." Cognitive reserve is built when people use their brains a lot: learning a musical instrument, reading difficult books or research articles, learning math and science subjects, and learning to speak other languages. Just like people can build muscle by lifting weights and exercising in a variety of ways, people can make more neurons and build cognitive reserve by exercising their minds.

The brain makes a lot of neurons in childhood. As we age, the production of neurons slow down. However, brain exercise can keep remaining neurons working AND can increase connections between neurons. This is also where a healthy diet and healthy lifestyle help with cognitive reserve. Just like we need to eat healthy food and get enough sleep to keep our bodies functioning, we need to do those things to keep the mind healthy.

The amount of cognitive reserve helps explain why dementia may look worse in one person compared to another. Vascular dementia can show up after decades of silent damage. Little bits of the brain are cut off from the blood supply and die off. Depending on how much "cognitive reserve" is present (Arnold versus Sheldon), the damage is not always as noticeable. The person's memory is fine, he or she is working and productive, life is great. At some point, however, the damage builds up until the brain can no longer compensate or adjust to the changes. Then, you begin to see signs like short-term memory loss, repeating the same questions repeatedly, and trouble finding words.

Vascular Dementia and Alzheimer's dementia

The changes in memory and ability to do things can be similar in both diseases. To make it even more confusing, a person may have both vascular dementia and another type of dementia together, such as Alzheimer's dementia. Some experts believe that the cardiovascular (heart and blood vessel) damage brings on the memory loss from Alzheimer's disease (or another dementia) sooner than if the person had never had any cardiovascular disease.

Dementia with Lewy Bodies [Lewy Body Dementia, Parkinson's Disease Dementia]

"Lewy Bodies" are abnormal proteins that show up in the parts of the brain the handle memory, sleep, movement, and "automatic" bodily functions like heart rate and blood pressure. Some people start out with difficulty moving and tremors and are initially diagnosed with Parkinson's Disease. Over time, they develop memory problems. In these cases, clinicians use the term "Parkinson's Disease Dementia" to describe the illness. Other people start out with memory problems and then later develop movement problems. These people are given the diagnosis "Lewy Body Dementia" or "Dementia with Lewy Bodies." These diseases are really two sides of the same coin.

Lewy Body Dementia (LBD) can be tricky to diagnose, especially if the memory problems start first. The brains of people with LBD are also low in acetylcholine. Therefore they often respond well to traditional acetylcholinesterase (ah-see-tel-col-een-es-ter-aze) inhibitors like rivastig-mine (Exelon)—and why a diagnosis of Alzheimer's dementia may be given at first, until the other symptoms start appearing. Other symptoms that point to LBD include:

- acting out dreams

- confusion that seems to come and go

- problems with "automatic" functions like blood pressure control

- movement problems including falls and tremors

- hallucinations, or seeing/hearing things that others do not. Halluci-nations are usually visual and are not always disturbing to the person.

The Lewy Body Dementia Association has an excellent website with much more information. Check out www.lbda.org.

Frontotemporal Lobar Degeneration/Frontotemporal Degeneration/Frontotemporal Dementia

Frontotemporal dementia (FTD) looks much different from the other de-mentias. Strange behaviors usually arrive before the forgetfulness. FTD tends to show up in people in their late 40s to early 60s, a time when most of us are still working. The biological culprit is the tau (pronounced like "towel" but without the "l" on the end) protein. Tau is a needed building block for nerve cells, but for some reason, too much tau gets produced and the brain cells start to die off. The brain cell death is mostly in the frontal lobe (the part of your brain that sits behind your forehead) and the temporal lobes (the two sides of your brain that sit around your ears). These two places are your "adult" brain, the responsible pieces that force you to bite your tongue before making some smart-ass response to your boss, or giving you the motivation to delay gratification, like vacuum the floors instead of watching Netflix. These two places also house the behavior "brakes," also known as self-con-trol. The "brakes" keep you from eating an entire 5-pound bag of Halloween candy in one sitting or drinking an entire case of beer in two hours. I will talk more about the different parts of the brain and their unique jobs in Chap-ter 5.

FTD has several different "faces." Here are two. For more, go to the Association for Frontotemporal Degeneration website https://www.theaftd.org/.

- *Behavioral variant FTD (bvFTD)*. This is like losing the brakes a little at a time. The recall ability of the brain, the part that can tell you the date or repeat and recall 3 words during a memory test, behaves normally at first. The personality starts to change, and not in a good way. A loving and responsible spouse/partner starts visiting dating sites, neglects the bills, or both. A fitness fanatic stops going to the gym and begins to pig out on sweets. The financially responsible accountant begins to send money to obvious (to everybody else) scammers. These behaviors often start out in small, sneaky ways and finally become too bizarre to ignore. It is not unusual for persons affected by FTD to come to the neurology clinic by way of law enforcement.

- *Primary progressive aphasia*. This "face" also has several subtypes as well. The person loses the ability to speak in a way that makes sense. Sometimes, the person loses the ability to retrieve categories of word like nouns. So the sentence, "The cat ran under the table when the dogs came into the room" may sound like "The...you know, the thing, it has whiskers, it ran under the...um...the thing, you put things on it..." Other people can speak without difficulty but their words make little sense to the listener, "The catch loped over the trauma when elephants sat down." Some individuals are so badly affected that they become unable to speak at all.

FTD does not usually respond to the medications commonly used with Alzheimer's dementia. In fact, such medications can make the behaviors much worse. These individuals usually respond better to rewards than negative consequences. Some of the behavioral techniques in this book can be used to deal with refusals.

Caregivers of persons with FTD may feel frustrated in support groups where most caregivers are dealing with Alzheimer's demnentia. Also, the cost of caregiving for a person with FTD is much greater than the financial cost of caring for someone with AD. Therefore caregivers dealing with FTD would benefit from their own support groups and Facebook pages. It IS different.

Bottom Line

Many of the behaviors that family and formal caregivers deal with are present regardless of the type of the dementia. While it is good to know what type of dementia you are dealing with, because some medications are better for one dementia over another type of dementia, it does not really matter when you are dealing with behaviors. Throughout this book, I will alert you if a technique or strategy should be adjusted for a specific type of dementia.

▪▪

Want more support and assistance beyond this book? Contact me about group and private options: rita.jablonski@gmail.com!

CHAPTER 2

Memory Problems that May Not Be Dementia

Earlier in my nurse practitioner career I worked for a geriatric practice. This practice provided primary care to people residing in nursing homes. I admitted a woman from the hospital with a diagnosis of dementia. The first thing I did was look over her medications. Holy shit! She had been prescribed multiple medications that all slowed down brain functioning. As I looked over her history, I immediately knew what had happened. She had been living independently and developed pneumonia. She became sick enough to need hospitalization. While in the hospital, she developed a problem called delirium (more on that later in this chapter). The physician overseeing her care mistakenly diagnosed dementia, which is a common occurrence. She must have been a bit feisty at the hospital because she was prescribed benzodiazipines (drugs like Xanax or alprazolam) and some serious antipsychotic medication. No wonder she was confused!!!

The first thing I did was stop 80% of her medications. Two weeks later, she was showing less confusion. Within 2 months, she showed no memory problems. Her family claimed that I had "cured" her dementia and treated me like a miracle worker. Nope. I successfully treated her delirium and removed a ton of pharmaceutical crap. She never had true dementia.

In fact, memory problems can be caused by a multiple of problems and medicines. This is why there are people all over the internet claiming they have "cured" dementia. The majority of these claims are outright horseshit. Pure fucking scams. A few of these claimers likely did what I did—fixed a fixable problem—except these claimers have no idea what a delirium is.

One of the annoying things about social media is that if you are a family caregiver for someone with dementia, regardless of type, well-meaning family and friends will start tagging you every time they encounter a dementia "cure." You may find yourself wanting to try all sorts of things to cure your loved one. That is understandable. Please be assured, that as of 2021, there are NO cures for dementia. If anyone advertises that they "cured" dementia, they are WRONG. If the person claiming to have cured Alzheimer's dementia or some other dementia is a healthcare provider, run. This person should know better, and if they do not, you do not want to be trusting your care to them. If the person claiming is friend or family caregiver, they mean well but were fooled by one of the **dementia fakers—other health or substances that can cause REVERSIBLE memory loss.**

Here are some culprits that can cause memory problems and are sometimes responsible for an incorrect diagnosis of dementia, especially in older adults:

Depression/Anxiety. Persons with depression can have problems with memory retrieval and completing activities that require thinking. There is some controversy, though. If the memory problems are mild then treatment with an appropriate medication may improve memory performance. On the other hand, there is some emerging evidence that people whose brains are starting to change due to dementia may be more sensitive to becoming depressed. That is, the depression is an early-warning sign that neurons are dying (neurodegeneration); the depression is really "unmasking" the dementia.

Low oxygen levels (from sleep apnea, lung problems, or anemia). Neurons, or brain cells, need oxygen to function. If there is not enough oxygen getting to the brain because of sleep apnea, not enough red blood cells to carry the oxygen (anemia) or lung disease, you will see more confusion and memory problems.

Poor blood flow to the brain. If blood is not getting to the neurons, neither is oxygen (see above). Poor blood flow can be causes by a variety of medical problems (low blood pressure, abnormally low heart rate, or unusual heart rhythms [atrial fibrillation]).

Medications. Some medications change the chemistry in the brain. Brain cells use certain chemicals, like acetylcholine, to make and hold memories. Medicines that interfere with acetylcholine levels can create temporary memory loss. Other medications, like dapsone, can interfere with oxygen getting to the brain. Narcotics, certain seizure medications, and a class of drugs known as benzodiazepines (drugs like Xanax, also known as alprazolam) cause slow mental functioning.

Thyroid problems. The thyroid gland, located in your neck, is the thermostat of your body. If the gland is not running up to speed, everything in your body slows down—including your thinking. People with low levels of thyroid hormone may also gain weight and be very sensitive to the cold. If the thyroid levels drop dangerously low, the person can go into a coma.

Artificial sweeteners. This is very controversial right now. There are links between certain artificial sweeteners, like aspartame, and headaches or migraines. Some people are just more sensitive to artificial sweeteners than others. I have a family history of sensitivity to artificial sweeteners, so I stopped using them.

Liver problems. The liver is responsible for breaking down medications and foods. If the liver is not working properly, some toxic substances stay in the body and tiredness and mental confusion can happen. There are usually other signs first, like a swollen abdomen, dark urine, light-colored stools, and lack of appetite.

Sleep Problems. The brain needs a certain quantity of quality sleep. Untreated sleep apnea can cause thinking and memory problems. Fatigue interferes with brain functioning. Sleep deprivation can cause the same level of impairment as heavy drinking!

Pain. Pain itself can cause memory problems because the pain becomes the focus of your attention and concentration. Opiates used to treat pain also cause memory problems.

Vitamin deficiencies. Low vitamin D can cause memory and thinking problems. Vitamin B12 can make existing memory problems much worse.

Delirium. This is a sudden onset of confusion that usually occurs during severe illness or hospitalization. Delirium can get better and worse, meaning it fluctuates, over the course of several hours. Once the illness is addressed and the person's health becomes better, the delirium USUALLY clears. It can take up to 3 months for some people. If an older adult without memory problems develops delirium, he or she may be at risk for developing dementia. Researchers believe that delirium in this situation means that the older adult has brain changes consistent with Alzheimer's dementia or one of the other dementias, but there has not yet been enough damage to cause observable problems. In other words, the delirium is "unmasking" the dementia. I explain more about delirium that happens with people who have dementia in Chapter 3.

If your loved one does have dementia, you can help keep their brain functioning at optimal levels by addressing all of the issues above.

Bottom Line

If you or someone you know is having problems with thinking and/or memory, the first place to start is the primary care provider. He or she should provide a thorough examination, check blood oxygen levels, and examine laboratory results. Depending on the results, the next step may be a neurology appointment for a more in-depth evaluation.

But what about claims that certain things "cause" dementia?

Sometimes, two events consistently happen together. This is called "correlation." I had a statistics prof who used to show the class an impressive graph comparing national ice cream sales with drownings. Both ice cream sales and drownings steadily increased in April, peaked in July, then slowly dwindled by October. Does this mean that ice cream eaters were more likely to drown than non-ice cream eaters? Nope. Both ice cream sales and drownings occur more frequently in summer months. Neither was related to each other. There are ways to show "correlation" mathematically, using statistics. But here is where it gets fun. Just because two things tend to happen together, it does not mean one is causing the other. As my statistics prof was fond of saying, "Correlation does not equal causation."

Researchers love to take large sets of data and look for correlations between life events, health problems, and Alzheimer's disease. One topic that seems to come up a lot is gum disease and dementia. In some correlation studies, gum disease and Alzheimer's disease follow the ice cream and drowning pattern. They exist together. I would not argue that dementia causes gum disease. HOWEVER, I know from my own research https://d.docs.live.net/f22286d80c8b00ac/MDYB%20Book/%22https:/o nlinelibrary.wiley.com/doi/full/10.1111/ger.12357%22%3eresearch that people living with AD and other dementias often stop brushing their teeth. They fight the efforts of others to provide mouth care. Without consistent mouth care, plaque builds up on teeth and along the gum line and soon, gum disease develops. The dementia did NOT cause the gum disease; lack of mouth care caused the gum disease. By the way, my team and I have tested a whole slew of ways to get people living with dementia to accept mouth care to fix this issue. You can click here https://www.ncbi.nlm.nih.gov/pmc/articles/PMC4861900/ to read the publication.

There are also some studies, again looking at correlations, that suggest that people with gum disease may be more likely to develop Alzheimer's disease and other dementias. One has to be careful here. People who develop gum disease usually have other health problems, like heart disease and diabetes. Some scientists have suggested that long-standing gum disease MAY cause heart disease. Other scientists have documented that diabetes and gum disease may aggravate each other. People with diabetes and heart disease are also at greater risk for developing dementia as they age. Diabetes and heart disease contribute to vascular dementia which IS preventable.

None of the dementias (Alzheimer's dementia, vascular dementia, Lewy Body, frontotemporal) are caused by one single issue. In fact, few people have just one type of dementia—many have at least two or more happening at the same time.

I am not suggesting that people simply say "screw this" and adopt a fatalistic attitude about their dementia risk. I am suggesting that there is more to the dementias than we know and understand... today. The take-home message is that one of the best ways to reduce dementia risk is to adopt a balanced and healthy life. We are social beings who need to belong. We are creative beings who need outlets. We are spiritual beings who need sacred spaces. If we engage less, if we stop meeting our many needs, if we stay stuck in unhealthy relationships (with people, food, booze, work, even medications) we jeopardize our overall health—and our cognitive health.

Bottom Line

These relationships (like many relationships!) are extremely complicated. Reporters who push exciting headlines are more interested in getting readers, not explaining the truth.

Is Memory Loss a Normal Part Of The Aging Process?

Maybe, maybe not. Once upon a time, poor physical health was considered a normal part of aging. It is not. Yes, there are aging-related changes but some of those changes have to do with lifestyle changes, not aging.

I hang with a tribe of fearless women who range from mid-50s to 80s. They hop on horses and take incredible jumps, fox hunt, and make that 2-ton horse prance like a ballerina in a dressage arena. We partner with these large, majestic creatures because we stay physically (and mentally) fit. And we are (mostly) adrenaline junkies. Some of our most athletic horses are geriatric equines—30+ years old—that are beating the odds because we take excellent care of them. The point is both the humans and animals in my world are defying stereotypes about aging and physical ability.

We can apply the same thinking to brain health. Yes, neurons do die off as part of the aging process. But we may make the process of neuron loss much faster!! If we slowly limit brain activity, more neurons die off from inactivity. Just like muscles weaken and shrink if not used, but tone and firm with regular movement and weight-bearing, the neurons respond to physical, mental, and social exercise.

Where Does Healthy Eating Come In?

Like the body, the brain needs fuel. The body is not designed to get nutrition from pills, but from whole foods. Eating brightly colored (and varied) fruits and vegetables, lean proteins, and plant fats have been shown over and over and over again to improve physical and mental health. Plus, there is the mind-body connection. If my body feels good (in part from good nutrition), my thinking feels clearer. I feel sharp. If my body feels bad, I cannot concentrate.

Here is where diet CAN fit in. Healthy diets increase blood flow to the brain. Healthy diets reduce the threat of diabetes. Healthy diets plus exercise reduce cardiovascular disease—less cholesterol (plaque) clogging up the arteries. Cardiovascular disease causes strokes, sometimes without symptoms. If you have enough small strokes in your brain, you lose memory and the ability to do activities over time. The memory problems from these strokes often show up as people age, because they are also losing neurons.

No "One Cause" Dementia

Bottom Line

By staying in our maximum state of physical, social, spiritual, and mental health, we can reduce many risk factors for dementia. If developing dementia is in our future cards, optimal health choices now may delay its appearance in our lives.

***

Want more support and assistance beyond this book? Contact me about group and private options: rita.jablonski@gmail.com!

CHAPTER 3

Dementia Stages

The journey through dementia is influenced by the type of dementia (like vascular or Lewy Body) and the person's personality and physical/mental health, to list just a few items. These stages are rough categories. People living with dementia will not always fit "neatly" into a specific stage. There is also movement within each stage.

Mild Behavioral Impairment

Many families of persons living with dementia have reported changes in personality, work habits, sleep, appetite, and even unusual aggression or anger that happened in the person's fifties, and occurred years before any memory changes were noted. In fact, the original patient treated by Dr. Alois Alzheimer had emotional problems and delusions that her husband was cheating on her well before she started having the memory problems that caused her family to seek help.

Dr. Ismail Zahinoor and colleagues published the Mild Behavior Impairment Checklist in 2017[1], and researchers continue to use these checklists in

---

[1]Ismail Z, Smith EE, Geda Y, et al. Neuropsychiatric symptoms as early manifestations of emergent dementia: Provisional diagnostic criteria for mild behavioral impairment. Alzheimers Dement 2016;12(2):195–202.

studies that may help us to better identify persons likely to develop dementia. The current thinking is that mild behavioral impairments can happen before mild cognitive impairment or simultaneously. This is an area that is continuing to be studied.

Mild Cognitive Impairment

Mild cognitive impairment (MCI) is a change in thinking or memory that can be noticed by the patient or another person (sometimes both). A clinician can find evidence of memory or thinking problems during an examination, which usually involves some type of memory testing. The person with the memory problems can live independently and may be able to work, depending on the type of job. Mild cognitive impairment is also known as mild neurocognitive disorder. Having MCI does not automatically mean the person will go on to develop a dementia. Usually, only close friends, family members, or colleagues notice that anything is "off."

Mild Dementia (2-4 years)

Sometimes this stage is known as "early stage" dementia. Dementia experts do not like to use the term "early stage" because it can be confused with early-onset dementia (dementia before age 60). People in this stage have episodes of forgetfulness and confusion. They may or may not report memory loss. People in the mild stage will frequently misplace familiar objects (like the TV remote or smart phone). Others may notice problems with using the correct noun. For example, instead of saying "cup," the person in the mild stage may say, "the thing you drink out of." People in this stage have difficulty remembering new material, like names of new acquaintances or using a new device (like an upgraded smart phone).

Moderate Dementia (2-10 years)

The person living with dementia knows his or her name, where they are currently located (such as the city of the doctor's office), and the day of the week and date. However, they are starting to need some help in order to safely live in their homes. They have problems with putting together tax paperwork, balancing bank accounts, and remembering appointments.

When persons living with dementia enter this stage, they may successfully compensate by using lists, calendars, notes, and alarms. As time goes on, they have more difficulty using these items and strategies. They start having problems dressing appropriately for the season and weather. Many become overwhelmed in new environments because they are unable to filter out unimportant sights and sounds and to pay attention to one conversation. They are unable to remember their date of birth and current address. When asked where they live, they may provide a location from decades ago.

Family caregivers often ask me, "is it safe for people in this stage to be left alone?" It depends. Can the person living with dementia recognize a threat (like a kitchen fire) and safely exit the home? Call 911 if they fall and are hurt?

Severe Dementia (1-3 years)

People with severe dementia cannot live independently. They require partial or full assistance with basic activities like dressing, bathing, toileting, and eating. They may talk much less, or not at all. They usually become bedridden.

Factors That Affect Time in Stages

The duration for each stage is an average and depends on many factors:

- Overall physical and mental health. People in excellent health with few other diseases may remain in MCI or mild for much longer than people with heart disease and past histories of strokes. Diseases that affect blood vessels in the brain (like high cholesterol, which increases risk for strokes) reduce blood flow to brain cells and the cells die.

- Cognitive reserve. Remember Arnold and Sheldon from Chapter 1? People who have built up their brains have created a large number of neurons and connections between the neurons. These people can experience much more brain damage before showing signs of dementia.

- Lifestyle changes. Any positive lifestyle change, like more exercise and better eating, reduces risks for other diseases that cause brain cell death. Weight loss, for example, can improve blood pressure and blood sugar, and result in better brain health.

- Quality of care. Persons living in environments where they are stimulated mentally, emotionally, physically, and socially do better than those who may be isolated, or who live with caregivers who are unable (or unwilling) to provide healthy environments. Just like everyone can sing but not everyone is a singer, not everyone has the ability to be a caregiver.

Sudden Changes in Memory, Abilities, and Behaviors

A sudden worsening in memory or sudden increase in behaviors can not be ignored. Something else is going on that is stressing out the brain and causing a problem called *delirium*. In Chapter 2, I described delirium, which is often mistaken for dementia in older hospitalized adults. A lot of caregivers do not realize that delirium can happen "on top" of dementia.

People living with dementia already have problems with memory and function. If people living with dementia get sick, let's say with a bladder infection, the body has to move resources to deal with the illness. It would be like a town that experiences damage from a hurricane and is functioning at 50% of normal, and then another hurricane arrives and creates more damage. Now the town is functioning at 25% of normal.

The biggest sign of delirium in a person living with dementia is more-than-usual confusion that happens suddenly. They may have NEW trouble walking or standing. They may start wetting themselves. They may become more angry and agitated, and try to strike their caregiver. Or they may become very sleepy and hard to awaken. In some cases, people can experience hallucinations or delusions. But the main way to tell apart delirium from the usual progression of dementia is THE SUDDENNESS OR ABRUPTNESS of the changes. As in, "Monday she was fine and by Wednesday she was so much worse."

When you see a sudden change in your loved one, think "delirium." And get them to a provider ASAP to figure out the cause! **PEOPLE LIVING WITH DEMENTIA ARE AT HIGH RISK FOR DELIRIUM!**

Why? A person with dementia is already struggling to think and to move. Using the hurricane analogy I used earlier in the chapter, the brain is like the poor town that gets hit with two back-to-back hurricanes—the town is overwhelmed and temporarily backslides. Another way to think about delirium and dementia is that the brain is a lot like an office or business in which half of the workers have been laid off. If a new problem shows up, the remaining workers become overwhelmed and cannot handle the problem. When something new shows up in the body that creates another problem, the body has to move resources to handle the problem, stressing the brain cells even more. The result is a temporary and sudden spike in confusion: delirium.

Infections are the usual suspects for delirium. Bladder infections are a biggie when it comes to delirium. But colds, the flu, and pneumonia can also trigger delirium. Other causes include:

- Overactive or underactive thyroid gland
- Medications
- An imbalance in certain important chemicals in the body, known as electrolytes
- Severe pain
- Constipation

Bottom Line

If you suspect delirium, act on your suspicions! Do not accept, "Oh, it is just dementia getting worse." Take your loved one to their primary care provider and have them examined. At the very least, check for a bladder infection.

CHAPTER 4

Meet the Brain

Dementia causes brain damage. It helps to have a basic understanding of the distinct parts of the brain, so that you can understand why certain behaviors happen.

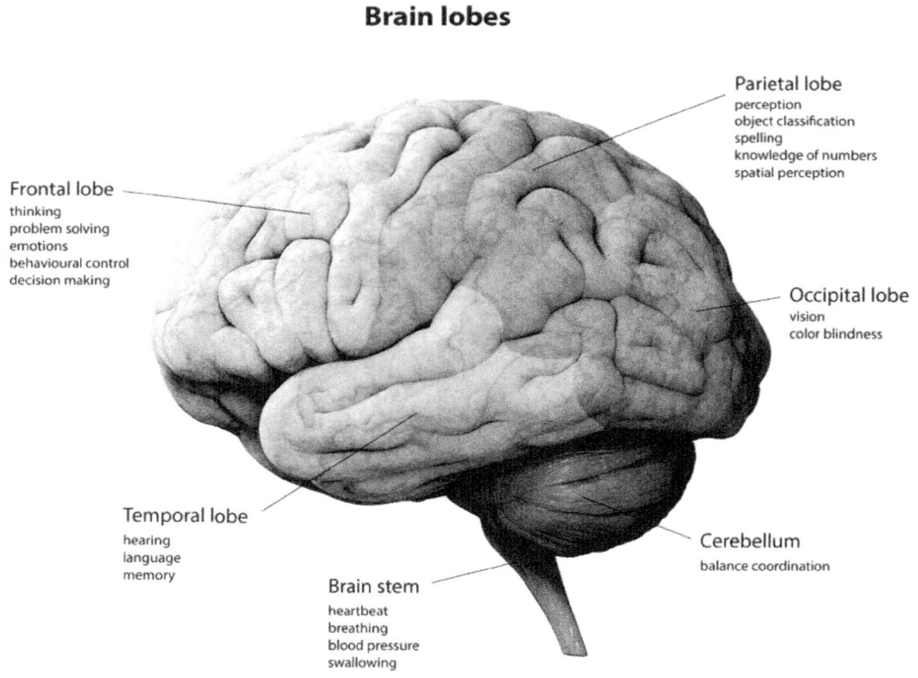

Brain lobes

Parietal lobe
perception
object classification
spelling
knowledge of numbers
spatial perception

Frontal lobe
thinking
problem solving
emotions
behavioural control
decision making

Occipital lobe
vision
color blindness

Temporal lobe
hearing
language
memory

Brain stem
heartbeat
breathing
blood pressure
swallowing

Cerebellum
balance coordination

Figure 1: Brain Anatomy and Functions

The brain above is a sideview. Imagine the person is standing in front of you but the person is standing sideways, facing the left side of the page. As you can see in the picture above, each part of the brain has its main "job." You are looking at the left side of the brain. The right side has the same lobes. You have 2 frontal lobes (right and left), 2 temporal lobes (right and left), 2 parietal lobes (right and left), and 2 occipital lobes.

This refers to the type of dementia and what parts of the brain are showing the damage. In all of the dementias, nerve cells in the brain are dying. The dying cells cause the brain to shrink. When a clinician looks at an MRI, they can see what parts of the brain are shrinking. This is also helpful when a clinician is trying to diagnose the type of dementias. Knowing what kind of dementia a person has can be helpful in selecting and modifying strategies, because distinct parts of the brain have specific jobs.

Let's take a look at the distinct parts of the brain and their jobs.

Frontal lobes are the part of the brain behind the forehead, also known as the "adult" part of the brain. The frontal lobes handle personality, social behaviors, and judgment. There is a section of the brain that sort of crosses both the frontal and temporal sections that is in charge of initiating action. When this part of the brain shrinks, the person starts to act like they do not give a shit. They becomes apathetic (ah-pah-thet-ic)—they seem to have no motivation and just want to sit on the couch and veg.

Temporal lobes handle understanding and making speech and remembering information that is heard—including music and sounds. The temporal lobes can be thought of as sound dictionaries. When I hear a word, the temporal lobes immediately link that sound to a word in the sound dictionary. The same thing happens when I hear a cat's meow—the temporal lobes take the sound information from the ears and link it to the word "cat." All of these linkages happen so quickly, you do not realize all of the steps involved!!

Parietal lobes help the body to identify sensations and to know where body parts (like hands, feet, arms and legs) are at all times. This is the part of the brain that helps you to tell the difference between a soft washcloth and sandpaper just by feeling the two, even with your eyes closed. The parietal lobes help us to classify objects (that is, we know a cat is an animal), understand the meaning of numbers, and spell.

Occipital lobes help the brain to identify what the eyes are seeing. These lobes work like the temporal lobes, except with pictures. The eyes send images to the occipital lobe, and the occipital lobe tells the brain what the picture means. This part of the brain is especially important for judging distances and understanding how two or more objects are physically related to each other. That is, the occipital lobe helps me to walk through a room with a lot of furniture and not walk into anything. The occipital lobe also helps me to know whether or not a kitchen chair will fit under the kitchen table.

The lobes work together to get things done. As you read the words in this book, your parietal lobes are helping you to understand what you are reading. The parietal lobes are also working with the occipital lobes so that you can make sense of the pictures and diagrams in this book. Distinct parts of the brain are helping you to pay attention to what you are reading and to concentrate on the information. If you are hungry, tired, bored, have to pee, or if you keep getting interrupted…you will have trouble following along until you take care of those problems.

While there are lots of cool parts of the brain deep inside, I am going to talk about two parts that are important understanding many dementia-related behaviors. These two parts are inside of the temporal lobes: the **amygdala** and the **hippocampus.** The amygdala and hippocampi are needed to make memories. The hippocampi are particularly important for turning immediate information into long-term information. Because of the hippocampi, I can tell you at 11 am what I did since waking up that morning. The hippocampi help me to keep track of a conversation and to figure out the "context" of a situation: how important or unimportant something is.

Figure 2: Structures Inside the Brain

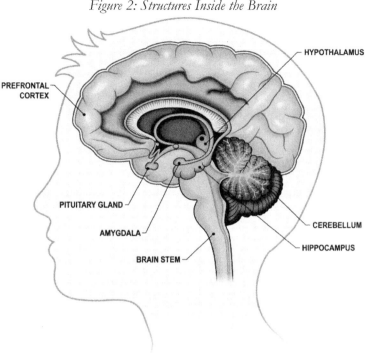

The amygdala is the seat of the fear response. It is the alarm bell of the brain. Another way to think about the amygdala is that is works like a smoke detector. The smoke detector goes off when smoke is around. The smoke detector does not tell you what is causing the smoke. When my smoke detector goes off in my house, I look around. Either dinner is ready or my sofa is on fire. Usually, dinner is ready. The amygdala tells the brain, "there is trouble." It sounds the alarm. The other parts of the brain, especially the hippocampi, figure out if the trouble is real and then the body goes into the fight or flight response. Or, the other parts of the brain tell the amygdala everything is OK and the brain quiets down.

Have you ever walked into a dark room and were startled because a strange man was standing in the room? And then you suddenly realize that you are looking at a lamp? Or, have you ever watched a scary movie and "jumped" when a character came out of nowhere? Once your brain realizes the threat is not real, you feel immediate relief. You may even laugh. The "startle" response is the amygdala and other parts of your brain working together to protect you.

When people have dementia, certain parts of the brain shrink—especially the hippocampi, which help the amygdala to tell the difference between something that is really a threat and something that is not. This means that persons with dementia are more likely to become fearful and see danger in **non-threatening situations**. Also, they have difficulty recognizing emotions: they are better able to recognize positive emotions rather than negative emotions, which explains why persons with dementia are **less likely** to resist care from smiling caregivers than from non-smiling caregivers.

Bottom Line

Some of the necessary care we try to provide to our family members with dementia may be accidentally scaring them. The changes in their brains make it difficult for them to tell the difference between a helping action and a harming action. This information will help you understand how and why the strategies I present in Chapter 9 (Preventing and Managing Care Refusals) work!

***

Want more support and assistance beyond this book? Contact me about group and private options: rita.jablonski@gmail.com!

PART 2

Understanding How
Brain Changes Cause Behavior and
What to Do About It

In 2018, I wrote a blog called "The 10 Commandments of Dementia Care." Since then, I have moved away from "commandments." I prefer to think of these as the framework or model for approaches to dementia caregiving that respects the personhood of the person living with dementia. I also am sensitive to the large numbers of caregivers who do not follow a Judea-Christian spiritual path (including me). This framework will help you shape your approach to dementia caregiving.

I. **I am still me.** I may forget parts of my life but I will never forget that I am an adult deserving dignity. Neither should you. My memories may go but my personality stays

II. **Treat me like an adult.** My behavior may be child-like, but NEVER treat me like a child. No baby talk!

III. **Come into my world, I can't function in yours.** This means that I can't remember what happened 5 minutes ago but I can remember something from 50 years ago. Please don't argue with me, I don't understand why you are angry and I feel terrible for hours afterward.

IV. **Actions are better than words.** No big explanations, a gentle touch or hug, and a warm smile goes a long way.

V. **Give me a daily, consistent schedule.** Consistent schedules tap the memories that I have and strengthen the parts of the brain that are still working. I feel better with schedules, even if I cannot remember them.

VI. **Give me nature.** I need fresh air and sunshine. Please make sure I get out every day, even if it is on a porch or patio, or near a big bay window, where I can watch the birds.

VII. **Give me pleasurable activities.** I may forget that you took me out to lunch, or we went fishing, but the pleasurable feelings and emotions that came from that experience will last for hours.

VIII. **Give me social interaction on my terms.** I can't handle large gatherings but I can visit with a couple of people, especially if they are following Commandment #3. Again, I may forget that the grandkids came to visit, but the pleasurable feelings and emotions from that visit will persist hours after the visit.

IX.   **Keep me safe.** That means giving me the freedom to move about my home as much as possible without falling or getting hurt. You may need to be creative, like hanging pictures of a bookshelf over a door to keep me from leaving.

X.   **Keep me healthy.** Help me to eat good foods to stay as healthy as possible, and help me to avoid infections.

CHAPTER 5

A Word About behavioral-variant Frontotemporal Dementia (bvFTD)

The next several chapters provide explanations for many dementia-related behavioral problems. These problems are presented in a general sequence that is (usually) seen in Alzheimer's dementia, vascular dementia, and dementia with Lewy bodies. bvFTD is very frustrating because it does not "play by the rules" and there are few resources out there for family caregivers. Perhaps there is a need for a book just for FTD caregivers called "Make FTD Your Bitch."

How Common is Behavioral FTD?

This dementia can show up in people who are in their 30s and 40s, although the majority of the cases show up when people are in their 50s. In fact, FTD is more common than Alzheimer's dementia for persons younger than 65. Research shows that the financial costs of caring for someone with FTD https://makedementiayourbitch.com/2017/10/18/frontotemporal-dementia-caregiving-costs-more-than-ad-caregiving/ is twice as high as caring for a person with Alzheimer's dementia. In my humble opinion, the psychological and emotional costs are probably much higher, too.

Behaviors First, Memory Loss Second

As I described in Chapter 4, the brain "shrinkage" that happens in bvFTD follows a different pattern than the other dementias. The frontal lobe usually starts to shrink first, quickly followed by the temporal lobes. There are individual variations, but you get the general idea. The front part of the brain is the "adult" brain and contains self-awareness and self-monitoring. This is the part of the brain that helps me to eat broccoli instead of M&Ms or get up and go to work when I would rather lay under the covers. The frontal lobe helps me to be a mature and responsible adult, not a jerk. People with mild bvFTD show problems with social comportment (that is, how to behave appropriately in social situations, like not using the F-bomb during a religious service), recognizing other people's emotions, empathy, and judgment. This is so frustrating for family members because this once awesome person is now acting like a major jerk. Meanwhile, he or she can easily breeze through traditional memory screening tests because these "office" or "bedside" screening tests really do not test executive functioning. It is no surprise that people living with bvFTD get in trouble at work, have run-ins with law enforcement, or find themselves in divorce court before a diagnosis is even made.

As the dementia progresses, short-term and long-term memory becomes impaired while apathy, hyperorality, utilization and stereotyped behaviors increase in frequency and magnitude. Functional abilities are lost in the reverse order they were learned. Language also declines; the person will begin to communicate using automatic phrases (for example, "How are you?" "I'm fine." "Things happen for a reason.") and then progress to mutism.

Personality Changes

One of the first "jerk behaviors" is more selfishness and lack of social etiquette. A warm, thoughtful, conscientious individual may begin to neglect spousal, parental, and workplace responsibilities. The individual may say or do uncharacteristic things in public. Family, close friends, and coworkers may notice the subtle changes but "brush off" the changes as stress, overload, substance abuse, or perhaps a "mid-life crisis."

Disinhibition and Impulsivity

These behaviors, coupled with personality changes, may result in behaviors such as gambling, sexual encounters, excessive shopping,

shoplifting, and traffic incidents. It is not unusual for a person with bvFTD at
this point to be fired from their employment or to have an encounter with law enforcement. In an interesting study by Liljegren et al (https://www.ncbi.nlm.nih.gov/pubmed/25559744), 14% persons with bvFTD compared to 2% of persons with Alzheimer's disease were found to engage in criminal behavior.

Apathy, Depression, Anxiety

Apathy, or "I don't care about anyone or anything," is from the shrinkage of an important piece of the brain known as the anterior cingulate cortex. Without the anterior cingulate cortex, people are incapable of feeling motivation and of performing activities in the correct sequence. The individual will completely lose interest in personal hygiene and will respond with "no" to any questions involving activity.

Hyperorality

When the brakes from the frontal lobe are gone, restraint disappears. Persons with behavioral FTD will constantly eat, especially sweet foods. Excessive smoking and drinking also occur. In my clinical practice, I have observed individuals resume smoking and drinking after stopping both behaviors decades earlier. As the disease progresses, these individuals may attempt to eat inedible objects.

Utilization and Stereotyped Ritualistic Behaviors

Utilization behavior refers to manipulating any and all objects in the environment or the "busy" person. A person with bvFTD will walk over to the nurses' station and begin handling telephones, pens, cell phones, and any object within reach. Telling them "no" DOES NOT WORK because this is a compulsive behavior. ***Stereotyped ritualistic behaviors*** include repetitive behaviors such as rocking, tongue clicking, or hand tapping. These behaviors can also include vocalizations like whooping, hollering, or grunting.

How Should Caregivers Handle the Behaviors?

Address the Environment

Because judgment goes before memory, the person with behavioral FTD appears "normal" to others. It is tricky to remove their access to joint checking accounts and other financial resources. However, this step must be taken. One of the first actions is to remove access to financial records and resources immediately, before those assets disappear. This means changing computer passwords and getting a PO box (or having bills and important documents sent to an alternative address).

Get Legal Help ASAP

You will need assistance obtaining the appropriate power of attorney documents. It will be helpful to obtain letters from your lawyers (who will request letters from the neurologist) to your banking institutions instructing them to NOT authorize transactions initiated by the person with behavioral FTD. Credit cards need to be off-limits.

Driving

This is an issue unto itself. I've addressed driving in Chapter 20.

Ritualistic Stereotypical Behaviors and Utilization Behaviors

Honestly, these two behaviors drive many caregivers up the wall. Ritualistic stereotypical behaviors do not really respond to medications. Boredom makes these behaviors worse. Meaningful activities (see Chapter 14) can help reduce the ritualistic behaviors. Exercise also helps and improves sleep. Caregivers should provide "safe" articles for handling when faced with utilization behaviors. Examples include bean bags, plastic cups and dishes, plastic keys, and expired or used gift cards (to mimic credit cards). Some families have created a room that is safe and contains objects for manipulation to prevent the person with behavioral FTD from destroying the entire house.

Falls

As the dementia progresses, falls become an issue because the parts of the brain that control voluntary movement start to shrink as well. Removing clutter and throw rugs are good first steps. The individual may benefit from physical therapy. The physical therapist can teach family caregivers appropriate exercises to help the person with behavioral FTD maintain as much function as possible.

FTD Care Costs Exceed AD Care Costs

As I noted earlier, persons receiving a diagnosis of FTD tend to be younger than persons receiving an Alzheimer's dementia diagnosis. FTD is the most common dementia experienced by people under the age of 60. FTD removes people from the workforce at a time when they may be at the height of their careers and their earning power. Additionally, the caregiver spouse also suffers financially when he or she reduces his or her hours, turn down a promotion because of caregiving responsibilities, or hires paid caregivers.

Dr. James Galvin and colleagues just published a paper http://www.neurology.org/content/early/2017/10/04/WNL.0000000000 004614.abstract examining the costs of caregiving for people impacted by FTD and comparing their numbers to caregivers of persons with AD. Dr. Galvin and colleagues surveyed 674 caregivers of persons with behavioral-variant FTD, primary progressive aphasia, FTD with motor neuron disease, corticobasal syndrome, or progressive supranuclear palsy. The majority of the caregivers cared for a spouse with bvFTD. Of all the diseases on the FTD spectrum, bvFTD was the costliest.

Families experienced a loss in income anywhere from $15K to $50K annually. The loss in income was due to the person with FTD leaving the workforce, the caregiver reducing work hours or leaving the workforce, or a combination of both. In addition to the lost income, **the direct cost of caring for a person with FTD averaged $48K annually.** These direct costs included medical care, residential care, respite care, medical equipment/supplies, and paid home care from formal caregivers. Indirect costs, which included the unpaid care provided by family members and lost wages, averaged **$72K yearly. Other costs that were NOT included in these numbers included fallout from poor decisions by persons with bvFTD, such as bankruptcy filings, guardianship hearings, will revisions, court appearances for criminal or civil matters, and associated attorney fees for all of the above.**

The combined indirect and direct care costs associated with FTD averaged $120K annually, compared to the average annual indirect and direct care costs of caregiving for AD, $64K. The exception to this is early onset AD, which comprises 5% of AD cases and affects people under age 65. Early-onset AD most likely follows the same cost-pattern of FTD; however, the experiences of these family caregivers gets swallowed up by the other 95% of AD caregivers.

If there are children involved, the economic (and social) ramifications become even more complicated. It may be impossible to save for college when sizable chunks of income are being siphoned off for care. Adolescent and teen-aged children are often recruited to help with care-giving. While not necessarily an automatically bad thing, adolescent and teen-aged caregivers probably require additional education and support... items that are in short supply for adult caregivers.

While not addressed explicitly in the article, I know first-hand that the working spouse becomes caught in a "between a rock and a hard place" scenario when the FTD progresses and the individual can no longer be safely left alone. The caregiver may not be able to quit work, especially if health benefits are tied to his or her employment. The only options include adult day care (and many adult day cares are not sympathetic to or equipped to manage the behaviors exhibited by persons with bvFTD) or paid caregivers. Difficult decisions have to be made, like how to cobble together a network of paid and informal caregivers to provide the needed supervision (and not get fired in the process!) Even after the person with FTD dies, the economic consequences persist for the spousal caregiver: debt, lower retirement income (if the caregiver works less and makes less money, then less money is put away for retirement), and inability to retire (especially if 401k's and other retirement funds were used for caregiving costs).

Bottom Line

Dementias that occur earlier in life have greater financial impact on family caregivers than those dementias that occur in later life. I would like to see more employers recognize the devastation wreaked by these dementias and to be more supportive of employees who are family caregivers. FMLA is great, but it is a baby step. Flexible work schedules and pre-tax health savings accounts for caregiving expenses are two ideas that would make life better for family caregivers.

***

I have experience working with many caregivers of people living with bvFTD. Please reach out to me if you would like to have me, your own personal dementia nurse navigator! And check out the free videos I have on https://makedementiayourbitch.com/videos/

CHAPTER 6

What People Living With FTD Want You to Know

My inspiration for this section came from three wonderful people who had been diagnosed with behavioral variant frontal temporal dementia. Their families were struggling with the behaviors and worse, with judgmental attitudes from their communities. All three of the individuals with dementia had some level of awareness of how differently they were treated when out in the community. At the time of this writing, all have passed. Their words still echo in my thoughts... and I share them below.

Dear Friends and Family,

Here are 10 things a person with FTD wants you to know:

1.   I have a brain disease. I am still me. I have some memory problems, so I repeat myself. A lot. I forget things, like shutting the door or what year it is. Actually, I don't care what year it is. Not sure if that is me or the disease. I can no longer drive. Well, I CAN drive and I think my driving is just fine, but everyone else constantly fusses at me about driving. See? This disease has robbed me of my ability to grasp and understand my own weaknesses while accurately realizing my strengths.

2.   The disease can rob me of my words. I may either speak slowly and with difficulty, or fast and easily, but either way my words may not make sense. I may say "cat" when I mean "couch," or "truck" when I want to say "fork." The connections between my mind and my mouth are fraying and breaking down. Please do not correct me or laugh at me. If you pay attention, you may see patterns and learn my language.

3.   FTD makes me forgetful, not stupid. I am VERY AWARE of how differently I am treated—like I have this horrible, CONTAGIOUS disease. Yeah, the disease sucks but what sucks more is being shunned. My disease has destroyed the parts of my brain that, in the past, put "brakes" on my words and actions. And don't judge! Every one of you has had that moment where you blurted out something that was better left unsaid. Some of you may not have my disease, but your "brakes" seem a little light. Anyone who has ever blurted something out without thinking has done what I am doing, although I'm doing it on a grander scale.

4.   Be patient and forgiving with my behavior. If a person driving a truck that suddenly lost its brakes was involved in an accident, would you blame the driver? No? So don't pass judgment on me or my caregiver! We used to go out a lot with friends and do things. Not anymore. My poor spouse, who is completely alone caring for me, is afraid to take me anywhere because of how YOU will react if I say or do something odd. I want to come to church. I would love to eat out with friends. I miss visits from my family (I think they are afraid that they are going to get this disease because our mother and grandfather had it, so they avoid me to pretend the disease does not even exist). I think my spouse/caregiver would be more likely to take me places even everyone was more understanding.

5.   Reach out to us without fear. If you say something and I become upset, change the topic. I'll forget what you said anyway. The nice part about this disease is that it is full of second (and third) chances. Not sure about what to say to me? Try some of these:

- "Hi, how are you?"

- "Glad to see you."

- "That's a nice shirt/tie/dress."

- "I've missed you."

- "I'm happy to see you."

6.   When offering to help, please be specific and follow through. I think many of you really do want to help us. My spouse is a bit proud and does

not want to bother anyone. Not me, I'll come right out and say it. Here are some ideas:

- "How about I visit with your loved one while you go food shopping. Let's figure out a day and time this week."

- "I'm making lasagna on Wednesday. I can bring some other and we can have dinner together. Would that work?"

- "The gang wants to help out. How about this Friday, the girls take you out while the guys visit?"

7.   Understand my limits and be kind. A part of my brain is not working, so the rest of it has to work even harder. It's like working a shift where half of my coworkers are out with the flu; the rest of us have to work twice as hard so we are exhausted at the end of the day. Big, noisy crowds and too many people talking at once exhaust me and I get cranky. If you happen to see me in a large gathering, please sit with me somewhere toward the fringes. This way, I can enjoy the experience without being overwhelmed. Likewise, if my behavior is interfering with others' enjoyment, gently and kindly taking me to a quieter place preserves my dignity, too.

8.   No matter how many times I tell the same joke or repeat the same sentence, please act as if you are hearing it for the first time.

9.   Please forgive and understand my relaxed physical boundaries. My grasp of socially acceptable behavior is very loose. I may hug you after meeting you for the first time, or I may start to talk with your child in the grocery store. I do not mean any harm or disrespect. The part of me that desires connection is stronger than the part of me that knows restraint. If I am making you uncomfortable, please simply step back and let my caregiver know in a kind and gentle way: "Sorry, I am not a hugger."

10. Be my guardian angel. Now that you know that I have a brain disease, please look out for me. I may start to walk over to the bathroom and get lost and start to cry. Newcomers to our community may gossip about my behavior. Please be my strength and my rock. "For whosoever did this for the least of my flock, they did it for me."

This section is dedicated to all of the wonderful people I know with FTD and their valiant caregivers. I HEAR YOU and I hopefully captured your "wish list." Please print this section out and hand it out to everyone in your community. If you want to reprint this for a newsletter or church bulletin, please contact me for permission (rita.jablonski@gmail.com). Together, we are going to make FTD our b*tch!!

***

Want more support and assistance beyond this book? Contact me about group and private dementia coaching options: rita.jablonski@gmail.com!

CHAPTER 7

Understanding Memory Problems in Dementia

In this chapter, I dive deeper into certain behaviors that appear in the mild dementia stage and persist throughout the disease journey. You will see that I use a lot of analogies to help you understand this information. The take-home message here is that many of the behaviors you deal with as a caregiver are caused or ramped up by brain damage. Your family member is not trying to piss you off on purpose, even though it may seem like it.

People with Alzheimer's dementia and vascular dementia usually start out with short-term memory problems. Family members notice more SDQs (same damn question) and problems with recalling details of conversations. These problems may seem irregular at first, happening more on bad days and less on good days. As I discussed in Chapter 2, the person's overall health (including sleep, anxiety, and depression) can make existing memory problems seem better on good days and worse on bad days.

SDQs (Same Damn Question)

"What time is it?" asks the person living with dementia.

"Five seconds since the last time you asked!" fumes the irritated caregiver.

Questions asked repeatedly can tax the patience of the most easy-going caregiver. It is a behavior that many formal and family caregivers find upsetting. Plus, caregivers are completely mystified how their spouse or parent or adult child (yes, there are moms and dads caring for adult children with dementia) cannot remember what they were just told but can relate a memory from 30 years ago.

Like I explained in Chapters 1 and 4, brain nerve cells die off in Alzheimer's dementia and other types of dementia. The loss of nerve cells causes the brain to shrink. The medical term for shrinkage is "atrophy." In the picture below, the brain on the left is showing significant atrophy or shrinkage, compared to the brain on the right. Although the picture is showing how amyloid plaques kill off neurons in AD, the loss of neurons (regardless of cause) causes brain shrinkage.

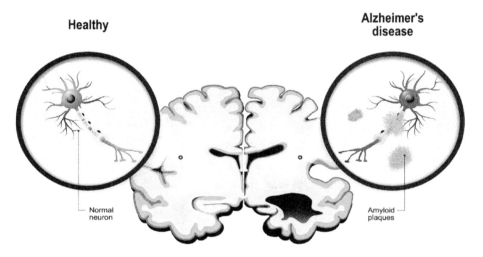

One way to think of a healthy brain is that it is like a box. All of your memories are placed in the box. Your earliest memories are tucked away in the bottom. Your most recent memories are on top. So, imagine your brain as a large box filled with all of your memories. What would happen if that box started to shrink, started to slowly become smaller?

That's right... as the box shrinks, the stuff inside falls out. The most recent memories, the ones at the very top, fall out first and are lost. This is why a person with dementia may forget what he or she had for lunch, or may even deny having had lunch at all. This also explains why people living with dementia can recall events from long ago so clearly. As the most recent memories fall out of the box, the memories that were buried are now more accessible. In fact, people living with dementia literally move backward in time. The memories from 40-plus years ago are now so vivid, they feel like they are reliving the memories, not just remembering.

If a box has shrunk, one cannot keep putting stuff into it. Likewise, as the brains of people living with dementia shrink, they lose the ability to make new memories. That is why your family member may ask you "What time is it" every 5 minutes, or revisit the same topic constantly during a 15 minute conversation. They are not trying to be difficult. They are making the most of what memories they are able to get to.

These same memory problems may show up as care refusals. In your family member's mind, he or she just bathed, even though you know he or she hasn't had a bath in 2 weeks. They may also be living in a time period of their lives when they had no health problems, so you handing them a bunch of pills does not make sense. What high blood pressure? As the dementia becomes worse, and the box shrinks even more, they may mistake a son or daughter for a spouse, or even fail to recognize a loved one. This lack of recognition can create more refusals. Would you let some stranger take off your clothes and stand you naked in a shower? I will cover strategies for care refusals later in this book in Chapter 9.

This brings me to a question I am constantly asked...

Do People Living with Dementia Remember what THEY Want to Remember?

Dementia can be puzzling to caregivers. Some short-term memories go "poof" while others stick around. Today, Mom cannot remember whether or not she took her medications, but she can tell you that YES SHE FED THE CAT! Sure enough, the medications are sitting in the little pill box but the cat is finishing up his breakfast. No, the person is not faking or being difficult.

Emotions can "Charge" Memories

When the memory starts to go, problems are first seen in the short-term arena. The person forgets some conversations as soon as they happen. This is the "shrinking box" phenomenon I mentioned earlier in this chapter. What confuses a lot of caregivers is that some short-term memories seem to stick around, while others fade away like candle smoke. The anchor that keeps some short-term memories alive while others literally go "poof" is **EMOTION**. What I just ate for breakfast, or the boring conversation (to me) I just had with my adult daughter, evaporates like a drop of water on a hot parking lot. But something with a lot of emotional voltage, like the damn doctor telling Dad he can't drive anymore, is going to anchor that new short-term memory in Dad's brain. If this event upsets him enough, he is going to bring up the topic repeatedly... causing his family to wonder, "I thought he had trouble with his short-term memory?? When is he going to forget about driving???"

Another way to think about this is go back to the shrinking box analogy. If I am determined that I am going to fit 25 pounds of shit into a 10-pound bag, I will use all of my strength to violate multiple laws of physics and MAKE 25 pounds of shit get into that 10 pound bag. Pretty much what I do when I cram a week's worth of clothes into a carry-on bag at the airport! If a memory is associated with enough emotion, if the voltage is high enough, the remaining neurons will respond to the emotional charge (good or bad, doesn't make any difference) and will burst out just enough brain juice (acetylcholine) to pin that memory into long-term storage.

This is why a person with dementia may go on and on (ruminate) about something that just happened but still be unable to tell you if they ate something for breakfast. The recent event is linked to a strong emotion, either positive or negative. The emotion "charged" the memory.

Caution: Negative Emotions

Unfortunately, negative emotions can also create and anchor memories. I have learned this the hard way. When I first began practicing as a nurse practitioner, I thought I had to administer a memory test at every appointment or I was not doing a decent job. One lady in particular became extremely anxious and tried to leave the examination room. Her family shared that it was becoming more difficult to get her to the appointments because of "the questions." Even though this lady had zero short-term memory, my actions triggered very strong negative emotions. These negative emotions "fired up" the remaining nerve cells, which processed the memory. She made a recent memory about her yucky experience and could now retrieve it. The good news is that I changed my approach and avoided triggering her anxiety.

She still was not happy about the appointments with me but she stayed in the room and seemed calmer.

Memories in Alzheimer's: Gone or Not Accessible?

"Will my mother forget who I am?" I receive this question, or variations of it, daily in my work with Alzheimer's patients. It is a hard question to answer. Some memories do become "erased" when nerve cells die. Other memories become hard to reach. Memories are like a washed-out road. I can see the road, and my destination, on the other side of the gaping, giant hole. I may see a detour. Awesome, I can get to my destination, but the detour may take hours and add miles to the trip.

In a healthy brain, pieces of a memory are stored in different places in the brain. Let's say I am enjoying a family dinner with my kids. I am making memories of this fun family dinner. The visual pieces are stored in the back of my brain, memories of the conversation is stored in the temporal area, and the delicious smells go into their special compartment. The overall emotions of love and happiness thread this memory pieces together, like beads or pearls on a string. Several weeks later, I smell roasted chicken while walking through the deli section of the grocery store and BAM! The aroma is identical to the roasted chicken I made. The recall of that aroma "tugs" on the aroma already stored in my brain and associated with the happy family dinner, and the whole memory "string" gets pulled out so that I can enjoy this happy memory.

If I develop dementia, a piece of the memory string may be cut off. The pieces of the memory are there, I just cannot get to them. When I try to recall the happy family dinner, I may only be able to get to one small piece of the memory: I remember my son being there, but not my daughter. Should I share this altered memory with my adult children and omit Sara, she may think that I have "forgotten" her. Nope. My memory of her is still in my brain, but the road getting me to my memory of Sara has been washed out.

Getting Around the "Washed Out" Road

Family members often try to "help" the person with dementia by telling them, reasoning with them, or even arguing with them about the correctness of a memory. If my daughter, Sara, were to argue with me and tell me she was present at the family dinner, this will only get me terribly upset. I would not forget my own daughter!! How silly! But I don't realize that my memory road is disconnected. That my memory string has been cut. Well-meaning family members and friends who try to convince the person with dementia about a specific memory are basically trying to get to the other side of the damaged road by driving into the hole. Nobody wins, nothing gets accomplished, and someone gets (emotionally) hurt.

This is where the detour comes in. Using the same scenario, my son decides to reminisce with me. Mark shares that he remembers a song on the radio that was playing while we were eating dinner. He hums a few bars of the song. That song tugs a different memory string, and as I follow the string, I wind up getting to the cut-off memories of that memorable dinner. Suddenly, I recall that Sara was singing along with the song as she and Mark cleaned up. Mark helped me to find a detour and get to the memory of the dinner.

More Connections Equal More Detour Routes

What helps us to recall memories? Connections. Another way to think of connections is layers. One flimsy plastic grocery bag will rip if I put a 10-lb bag of sugar in it. But if I use 3, 4, or even 5 plastic bags, all layered one inside the other, I can easily carry a 10-lb bag of sugar to the car without the bags ripping apart. The more nerve connections that are involved with the making of a memory, the more detour options I have to get to these important memories if I have a cluster of dead nerve cells (or neurons) in parts of my brain.

When I lived in rural Pennsylvania, I had one option to get to work: Route 322. There were other routes but they did not intersect, or connect with, route 322 for miles. A major truck accident would result in being stuck on route 322 for hours, something that occurred with annoying frequency during winter snow storms. In contrast, when I lived in Philadelphia, I had several alternate choices because of the busy grid of roads, highways, and interstates. Some of the detours took longer and were less convenient and direct, but I had options to arrive at my destination in spite of accidents or closed sections of highway.

Physical exercise, sufficient sleep, healthy eating, minimal alcohol consumption, and mentally-stimulating activities promote plentiful nerve connections. This is something we can all do now to help support our brain health and memories as we age. These same things can help maintain the connections already present in the brain of a person with dementia.

Brain Shrinkage Worsens Irritability

The brain is a lot like a business or company. Every brain cell is a worker and the parts of the brain are the different departments of a company. All of the departments must be staffed properly. In fact, the brain is more like a government bureaucracy—there is definitely overlap and redundancy! Redundancy is how the body protects itself from illness and damage. If one kidney is damaged, the other kidney picks up the slack. The brain is somewhat similar.

Using this example, imagine that the brain is a large government agency with multiple departments. You can pretend the different lobes of the brain are the different departments. The feds decide to trim the budget and eliminate 20 positions. Coincidentally, 20 employees are eligible for retirement, and they decide to leave. Once these 20 people head out the door and move to Florida, work resumes. Nobody feels any impact. The remaining workers easily absorb the functions of the retired workers.

This is sort of what happens when we age. The brain "prunes" away neurons that are not working or haven't fired in a while. Some neurons simply get old and die off. There are enough neurons to pick up the slack. No biggie.

A year later, and once again, 20 positions are eliminated. The same process happens every year. Some departments lose more positions than others. These departments become the obvious problem children and begin royally screwing up. Other departments run into problems because the problem children are not sending over the correct forms… or are not sending anything over at all!

The office compensates. The better staffed departments share their employees with the departments running with a skeleton crew. Even with these changes, any temporary loss of employees due to sickness or vacation makes it more difficult to function. During these times, there are more arguments, more blaming, more harsh words. Mistakes happen more frequently. A couple of customers notice that things aren't going as smoothly as possible, and a few comment that it is taking longer to get their orders done. Even though there are glitches, overall the office is meeting expectations.

A couple of months later, 20 more jobs are eliminated. All of the departments are short-staffed. The office has half of its original work force. Work quantity and quality drop. There is daily fighting, hourly disagreements, and continuous arguing. Fewer tasks are being completed correctly. Orders are wrong, projects are abandoned midway. Everything is a mess. Some employees become burned out and simply leave. When a quarter of the original workforce is left, the office is closed because it no longer has enough employees to run the office properly.

What I've just described happens in the brains of people living with dementia. Sometimes, the loss of nerve cells is sudden, like in a stroke. The majority of times, the loss of brain cells happens quietly over time, just like the gradual layoffs in the example above. A person with dementia has fewer brain cells trying to do the work of many brain cells. This explains why they are exhausted by the end of the day. This explains the frequent bouts of irritability or crankiness.

Mixed-Up Memories

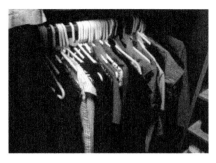

Another way to think of the brain is that it functions like a well-organized closet. You take apart an outfit and hang the shirt in one place, the pants or skirt in other section, and the shoes are organized in another section. When you need to put together an outfit, no big deal. You simply reach in and find the pieces that you want and put those pieces together. The pieces closest to the door are the easiest to get to, but you recall that nice wool jacket way in the back and you know to reach back and find it.

Your brain does a similar thing with memories. Each memory is like a piece of an outfit. Think of a good memory, perhaps a family vacation or winning an award. The images that are part of your memory go in one section of your brain. The sounds that make up that same memory are filed in the sides of your brain. Any sensations or tastes or smells that make up this memory you are having, those are all separated and filed in specific brain compartments. Your brain works similarly to a neat and orderly walk-in closet.

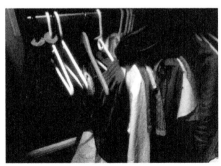

As cells die in the brain of a person with dementia, several things happen. First, the most recent memories are lost. Using the closet example, **notice the empty hangers in the left side of the picture**. They represent the lost memories. The items deeper in the closet, however, remain accessible. This is why persons with dementia may forget what you just told them or what they had for breakfast (or even if they have eaten), but they can tell you in detail something that happened in 1972. The memories that remain also get mixed up inside the person's brain. Notice that in the closet pictured here, there is a red pair of men's shorts and a solitary men's shoe mixed in with women's blouses; a white lab coat has also appeared in the shirt/blouse section.

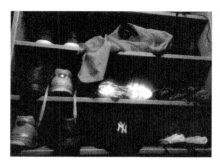

Remember how organized the shoes were? Now, some of the shoes are sitting next to the wrong mate, while a woman's pink blouse, a pair of silver heels, and some NYY baseball caps are residing where the shoes had been.

How difficult do you think it would be to put together an outfit from this disorganized and chaotic closet? How frustrated would you be if you went looking for your favorite black shoes and a pink shirt was sitting there instead? Or worse, what if you were unable to tell that the closet was all mixed up? What if you simply put together outfits based on what was available in the closet? You may wind up trying to use red gym shorts as a nice shirt (to be fair, it was in the blouse/shirt section) or using a baseball cap as a shoe (hey, it was there in the shoe section).

This "mixing up of memories" inside the brain of a person with dementia may explain why your family member might have trouble getting dressed in order, or may wear the same outfit repeatedly, or may argue with you that his or her outfit is appropriate. He or she is using available memories to function and to make sense of what is going on around him or her.

Some caregivers think they are helping their loved ones by "quizzing" them almost constantly and asking them to remember. There is a difference between helping someone with dementia process information with cues and hints, and treating them like they are a game show contestant. I will talk about ways to support a person's memory later in the book. At the same time, presenting logic and arguing does not work. It would be like me pointing to the empty hanger and telling you to put on the bright blue shirt—if your memory is like that second closet, you don't have a bright blue shirt and no amount of arguing will convince you otherwise.

Caregiver Vibes Influence Behaviors

We are energetic beings. Without even realizing it, we are advertising our emotional energy to the world. Some of us give off a lot of emotional energy. Some of us are a bit quieter.

We also absorb (or at least notice) other people's energy, their "vibes." Have you ever felt an immediate "like" or "dislike" of someone as soon as you both met? If your immediate response was a strong dislike, how did you describe that feeling? Did you say something like, "There is something about him/her that seems 'off'?"

Are there people in your environment that brighten up a room when they walk in? Do you know of others who do the same thing...when they leave?

In these situations, you are picking up on the energies of others, on their "vibes."

In the clinical setting, I use a tuning fork to check if a person can feel vibrations, especially if I am concerned about nerve damage from diabetes. This is because everyone has nerves which can feel vibrations and pass those vibration sensations up to the brain. I Even though we cannot hear or see those vibrations, we can still feel them.

Watch what happens when a vibrating tuning fork goes into a glass of water. https://youtu.be/YQtKf3qZHVs It happens so fast that the video makers slowed down the filming to show you what is really happening. Did you notice the water suddenly splash out of the glass? The vibrations from the tuning fork "agitated" the water.

Moods Can Be Contagious….Both Good and Bad!

So, what does this have to do with persons with dementia? People living with dementia, even if they cannot communicate verbally, can still pick up on caregiver "vibes" or moods. In other words, moods can be contagious: both good AND bad. If I'm in a good mood, my loved one may seem happy, calm, and cooperative. On the other hand, if I'm feeling exhausted or resentful or angry—even if these feelings have NOTHING to do with my family member with dementia—my loved one can feel agitated, just like the water became agitated. This unsettled or worried feeling may express itself as refusals or resistance to care.

CHAPTER 8

Dementia-Centric Communication

Dementia-centric communication is the ability to interact with people who have dementia in a respectful and meaningful way **that compensates for their memory issues**. The over-riding thing to keep in mind is that our communication patterns respect the dignity and personhood of the person with dementia. In other words, let me set you straight: the person with dementia is forgetful, NOT stupid.

General Communication Approaches

People living with dementia in the mild stage may start to notice that they have to work a lot harder to get the same things done. They may notice that they cannot tolerate places with a lot of people or noise. This is where family members notice that their loved ones seem to withdraw. They stop wanting to go out. They begin to avoid family functions because they know they will be overwhelmed. They may even withdraw from the caregiver.

It is Not Your Fault

As the brain loses neurons, the brain is unable to pay attention to important things when there is a lot of background noise. The remaining neurons must work super hard to do the tasks we take for granted. It is exhausting to try to follow a conversation, especially if the person living with dementia is already tired. Sometimes, the person living with dementia will fuss at the caregiver: "You ask too many questions!" "You talk too much!"

The caregiver is obviously hurt and confused, especially if the caregiver is really trying to adjust their communication styles. Here is what you can do:

SDQs (Same Damn Question): Always the First Time!

Treat every story, question, and anecdote as if you are hearing it the first time... because you are. If the person living with dementia asks you what time it is, you answer. And no, "Five seconds since the last time you asked" is not a good idea. The person living with dementia forgot that they forgot. Getting huffy and telling them that they told you this same story fifteen times will not work. To them, this is the first time they have told you this story or asked this question.

Dealing with Accusations

In this stage, people forget where they put commonly used objects. When my family member lived with me, she was always misplacing her wallet—which had her driver's license and Medicare cards. She would then tell me that one of my kids had stolen her wallet. I usually found it—she liked to put things under her pillow and between the seat cushions of her recliner. I finally gave her a wallet for her birthday (it was one of 4 identical wallets). I made multiple laminated copies of her driver's license and insurance cards and put the originals in my safe. I also collected old gift cards and put them in her wallet as credit cards. She still liked to shop, so I obtained a loadable debit card that I could give to her when we went out.

Adjust to their Best Times

People living with dementia may be at their best first thing in the morning, when there is plenty of "brain juice" swishing around the neurons. If you have an important topic that you need to discuss, this may be the best time. Other good times may be after a rest, like a short nap, or after a pleasant activity. When we engage in pleasant activities, our brains make more happy chemicals that also help reduce irritability.

Talk in a Quiet Place—for Real

Sometimes I call my son while he is working his night shift. I'm an early riser and 4 am is usually quiet, even for highway patrol. I suddenly hear his radio crackle and I immediately stop talking. "Go ahead, it's fine," he tells me. Mark can listen to me and filter out his radio because his brain is tuned to specific words and phrases. He has enough neurons to pay attention to our conversation and monitor dispatch.

I'm not that good. I find the radio very distracting. My brain has not been trained about what is important and what is not. I get to feel like a person with dementia because all of the crackles sound the same to me. In fact, if the radio is too busy, I find myself getting irritated and I end the conversation.

You may think you are in a quiet place because the background sounds do not bother you. There is a part of your brain that is hearing the fridge run, the radio play music, and the neighbor mow his grass. But your loved one with dementia is being pulled away by all of these sounds. Their brains are treating these "background" sounds as important messages. They cannot hear you... or they are having trouble focusing. It will help if you are sensitive to these sounds and make sure you and your loved on are in a truly quiet place.

Short, Sweet, Concrete

As I mentioned earlier in this book, the shrinking brain causes problems with both short-term memory and memory retrieval. The shrinking brain cannot handle lengthy explanations. We tend to speak in paragraphs. When talking with someone who has dementia, it is better to speak in bullet points. It is also better to keep the sentence structure simple. Compare these two directions:

- Before you turn on the light, make sure you close the door.

- Close the door. Turn on the light.

The second one is much clearer. It may feel really weird, but that is how to speak with someone who is experiencing mild cognitive impairment and mild dementia. The shrinking brain literally cannot "hold onto" too many ideas at once.

No Arguing, No Logic!

This is so hard for so many caregivers, probably because we have to un-learn lifetimes of communication styles. Arguing with a person living with dementia is pointless and you will wind up on an eternal hamster wheel. Logic also does not work, because they may not have enough available memory to follow the logic. Instead, they will likely become more angry and upset with you and you will both go down an exhausting rabbit hole. For example, daughter has just arrived at dad's house for his Friday morning doctor's appointment. The conversation goes like this:

Daughter: "Dad, you have a doctor's appointment today." *(Daughter has just arrived at Dad's house and is surprised to find him still in his pajamas).*

Dad: "I do? This is the first time I'm hearing about it." *(Dad really has no recall of this doctor's appointment. He feels surprised because he likes to know about things in advance).*

Daughter: "No it isn't! I've been telling you about this appointment every day since last Tuesday! I wrote it on your calendar, see? *(points to calendar hanging on fridge)* I even have all of these post-it notes all over the bathroom mirror *(walks to bathroom, points to mirror)*

Dad *(who only retained the last couple of words)*: "Yes, there are notes on the bathroom mirror." *(He walks over and starts to read the post-it notes)* "Doctor's appointment Friday, 9 am. I have a doctor's appointment on Friday?"

Daughter *(getting louder and more irritated, because now they might miss the appointment)* "TODAY IS FRIDAY! YOU HAVE A DOCTOR'S APPOINTMENT TODAY!"

Dad *(angry that his daughter is yelling at him for no reason because its not his fault she doesn't tell him anything. These emotions trigger old memories of his wife, who always missed appointments)*: "DON'T YOU YELL AT ME! I DON'T KNOW ANYTHING ABOUT A DAMN DOCTOR'S APPOINTMENT. You are just like your mother, she never remembered her appointments. *(pauses, starts to look around the house).* Where is your mother?

Daughter stops in her tracks. Her mother died 18 months ago. How does she handle this?

In the above conversation, several issues are going on. First, dad has little short-term memory. He is having trouble even with calendars and notes. He can read and understand the post-it notes but does not have enough memory for context, or to look at the calendar and figure out that today is Friday. He does have access to all of his emotions and he recognizes that his daughter is giving off serious vibes of anger and frustration. His daughter's emotions are triggering emotional connections to his wife, and he retrieves emotionally charged memories of his wife's tendency to forget appointments. Because of retrieval problems, he pulls out a piece of memory about his wife (who was terrible with appointments) but does not pull out the memory of her death. If given a few more minutes, that memory will likely follow and he will recall her death. The retrieval may take more time.

Daughter's use of logic and arguments are making a bad situation worse. She has to first abandon this approach and adjust her communication with her father. Another important strategy is to adjust her emotions. In the example above, the daughter's emotions (her vibes) were coming through. People living with dementia may have trouble following the words, especially as the dementia worsens. With the exception of bvFTD, they do remain sensitive to the energy of others. Nonverbal communication is also important. This is why it is a good idea to take a deep breath and smile prior to interacting with a person living with dementia. Any negative emotion, even negative emotion unrelated to the situation at hand, can poison the current interaction.

Anosognosia and Memory

In the first conversation between dad and his daughter, something called "anosogonosia"

(ah-no-soge-no-zi-ah) is happening. Anosognosia means that someone is not aware of their problems or disabilities. Many people living with dementia have no idea they have memory problems. They are unaware of what they can no longer do. Anosognosia upsets family caregivers. I see this in my clinic. The person living with dementia will tell me how they still cook family dinners or run the family business. Meanwhile, the family caregiver is vehemently shaking his or head "no"!

The person living with dementia is not lying! He or she has old memories of doing things—like making family dinners, taking vacations, cleaning out gutters, paying bills, and meeting friends for lunch. The loss of some memories combined with access to other memories creates this weird reality where it feels like they are still doing certain activities…even if you know that they are not.

The presence of anosognosia is another reason why arguing and logic are doomed to failure. I once had a wife ask me, at every appointment, to explain to her husband that he had dementia and he was unable to drive. She thought that her husband would listen to me because I was wearing the white coat. I gently told her that her husband did not feel like he had memory problems. I would only upset him, and she would have to deal with an angry spouse for the entire drive home. She then had the idea to record the appointment where I discussed his diagnosis of dementia. Reluctantly, I agreed. When she played the recording of the appointment for him later that week, he became very angry and upset: "There is nothing wrong with my memory." In fact, he became so upset that he created a strong, negative memory about the clinic (see "Emotions Can Charge Memories").

Apologize: I'm Sorry, I Forgot to Tell You…

This is an excellent technique to derail arguments and to get the person living with dementia back on (our) track. This is how the daughter could use the apology strategy in her situation:

Daughter: "Dad, you have a doctor's appointment today." *(Daughter has just arrived at Dad's house and is surprised to find him still in his pajamas).*

Dad: "I do? This is the first time I'm hearing about it." *(Dad really has no recall of this doctor's appointment. He feels surprised because he likes to know about things in advance).*

Daughter (*thinks about the multiple phone calls, the post-it notes all over the bathroom mirror, and the big red circle on today's date on the calendar hanging on the fridge. She takes a deep breath and calmly says*) "Oh, geez. I am so sorry. I forgot to tell you. You have a doctor's appointment today."

Dad (*starting to get angry*): You know I hate to miss appointments!

Daughter (*calmly*) "I know. I'm sorry. You go and get ready. I'll treat you to some coffee on the way."

The apology strategy works for a couple of reasons. First, it removes all of the arguing. Second, it takes the defensive feeling away from the person living with dementia. The caregiver may come off as "blaming" the person living with dementia, even if that is not the intent! If someone says to me, "I told you three times about X event," and I have no recall of this exchange, I immediately begin to feel defensive: "No you didn't!!!" I feel like I have to defend myself.

Putting It All Together

These strategies, coupled with some of the techniques I mentioned in previous chapters, form the foundation for dementia-centric communication. In earlier chapters, I explained how changes in the brain affected the way people living with dementia process and understand daily communication. These strategies help us, the caregivers, compensate for brain changes that affect the ability of the person living with dementia to understand and communicate with us. In upcoming chapters, I will provide strategies for care refusals and for other dementia-related behaviors.

CHAPTER 9

Preventing and Managing General Care-Refusal Behavior

As the dementia worsens and people living with dementia need more help, a weird thing happens. They begin to refuse the very help they desperately need. Care-refusal behavior can happen at any stage, but often begins during the moderate stage. In this stage, people living with dementia are unable to handle finances (this problem starts in the mild stage). They may be able to write a check, but may write it for the wrong amount, forget to mail it, or write duplicates. They are having more problems with cooking and other household chores. Because of anosognosia and mixed-up memories (remember the messy closet in Chapter 7?), they will "tell stories." People living with dementia are not lying. They are truly trying to rebuild memories with brains that have damage. This is the stage where people living with dementia need more supervision.

There are two main, general drivers of care-refusal behavior: The "automatic no" and refusals based on fear. The first part of this chapter will explain those two drivers. The second part of the chapter will describe strategies that you can use immediately to prevent care-refusal behavior. The last part of the chapter will describe strategies to help you manage care-refusal behavior as soon as it happens.

Section 1: Causes of Care-Refusal Behavior

Automatic "NO!"

People living with dementia towards the end of the moderate stage often say "NO" to nearly every question or request. This is an incredible challenge for caregivers. In this section, I explain one reason for the non-stop no's…and offer strategies for preventing and managing the negativity.

"Mama" and "NO!"

The earliest words uttered by babes are usually "mama" and "no." Any parent can relate to the "NO" word. "NO" is how we protect children from harm and teach them how to behave. Even if we make the home environment as safe as possible, "NO" remains important as our children get older and go outside into the world. They learn to use "no" to establish boundaries. "Just say no" and "No means no" are now embedded in our culture.

When the toddler first uses the word "no," he or she is not refusing anything. They are simply trying out their teeth and tongues, repeating this cool new thing they learned to do. When my youngest was learning to talk, and "no" was one of his earliest words, his older sister loved to tease him by asking him questions—knowing his response:

Older sister: "Want some ice cream?"

Little brother (*smiling and reaching for the spoon*): "NO!"

Older sister: "Sorry, little guy, you said 'no.'" (*Older sister puts spoon of ice cream in her mouth.*)

Little brother starts to cry and wail.

Mom: "DO NOT MAKE ME COME OVER THERE! STOP TEASING YOUR BROTHER!!" (and various other things that I probably should not have said but other parents will understand).

As adults, we continue to use the word "no." Sometimes, we use it to protect ourselves from negative choices: "No, I am NOT going to (make that purchase, eat that food, tell my supervisor she is a fucking idiot, etc.)."

Sometimes, we struggle to use the NO word to avoid being over-committed or to set boundaries, for fear that we may be disappointing others.

Bottom Line

Our use of the word "no" starts around the same time we are learning to feed ourselves with our fingers and is used multiple times a day throughout our adulthood and older age. The use of the word "no" eventually becomes a procedural memory. A procedural memory is the memory of how to do something. Procedural memories, which include feeding oneself and brushing one's teeth, will remain even after we lose other memories, like why or when we should do something. I go more in-depth about procedural memories in Chapter 14.

Dementia and "NO"

As people living with dementia move backward in time, it makes sense that the use of the word "no" remains. The ability to say "no" will be among the last memories and abilities lost by a person with dementia. Just like my example above, the knowledge of the meaning may go away even though the ability to make the word remains.

Beyond Yes/No Questions

When working with persons with dementia, we immediately learn NOT to ask yes/no questions. We change our tactics and say, "Time to take a bath," or "Here are your medications." The dreaded NO still happens. Why?

Too Many Words Not Enough Memory

People with worsening dementia can only "hold onto" a few words at a time. We often use sentences that are too long. Or we try to "explain" why medications are important. Logic and explanations do not work. There is not enough available memory to process this information. When the number of words are greater than the brain capacity, the brain falls back on the procedural memory of "no."

Shrinking **Temporal** Lobes Cause Problems Understanding Spoken Words

The temporal lobes (under the ears) shrink in Alzheimer's dementia and frontotemporal dementia. These same lobes are often damaged after strokes, which causes the receptive aphasia we see with post-stroke patients. The temporal lobes link sounds to words. As the temporal lobes shrink, people living with dementia no longer understand speech. In fact, I have observed that many people with moderate dementia start to act as if they have a hearing problem: "Huh?" "What?" "What did you say?" "I can't understand." The hearing works; the ability of the brain to pull the word out of the brain dictionary and link it to the sound is broken.

Our words, then, lose meaning. The result? Automatic "no."

Refusals Based on Fear

One reason why older adults with dementia resist care can be found in the human brain. We evolved with the ability to automatically respond to anything that could be threatening. This automatic response is the "flight, freeze, or fight" response that you first learned about in Chapter 4. For example, let's say you are driving your car down the interstate and the vehicle in front of you comes to a dead stop. Immediately, your body takes over—you simultaneously slam on the brakes while swerving to avoid the car in front of you. Your heart is furiously pounding and you seem to see everything in slow motion. Afterwards, it may take several minutes for your heart to slow back down to normal.

What I've just described is the automatic fear response. The fear response is governed by several parts of the brain known collectively as the limbic system or "lizard brain." The fear response has both autonomic pieces (fast heart rate, fast breathing, sweating) and behavioral pieces (freeze, flee, or fight).

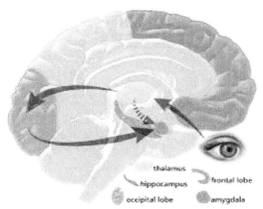

Figure 3: The Amygdala. Licensed under the Creative Commons Attribution 4.0 International License. https://commons.wikimedia.org/wiki/File:The_Fear_Processor.jpg

Using the driving example, when you saw the stopped car, the images traveled from your eyeball to the thalamus and amygdala (the yellow and pink circles in the drawing). The amygdala decided that this was a dangerous situation and it sent a signal right to your brainstem, which unleashed the automatic responses: the increased heart rate, fast breathing, and sweating. This allowed the rest of your body to respond to the threat by trying to avoid the collision—slamming on the pedals and swerving. You were trying to "flee" from a potential accident.

Now, let's talk about how your brain can tell the difference between something that is truly a threat and something that is not. Let's say I am afraid of spiders and one of my friends wants to play a prank on me. I go to my desk and see this big, nasty, scary spider. The same freeze/flee/fight response initially kicks in, but... I realize that the spider is a Halloween decoration! This time, other parts of my brain kick in—particularly the hippocampus (light blue swoosh in the picture above) and frontal cortex (blue-purple part), which "tell" the amygdala that the spider is fake and not a threat. Before the full flight/fight/freeze response can go into high gear, my brain calms down. I can now laugh at the situation and pick up the fake spider and use it to play a prank on someone else. This entire process takes nanoseconds, which means it feels immediate to you and to me.

When people have dementia, certain parts of the brain shrink—especially the hippocampi, which help the amygdala to tell the difference between something that is really a threat and something that is not. This means that persons with dementia are more likely to become fearful and see danger in **non-threatening situations**. Also, they have difficulty recognizing emotions: they are better able to recognize positive emotions rather than negative emotions, which explains why persons with dementia are **<u>less likely</u>** to resist care from smiling caregivers than from non-smiling caregivers.

Bottom Line

Some of the necessary care we try to provide to our family members with dementia may be accidentally scaring them. The changes in their brains make it difficult for them to tell the difference between a helping action and a harming action.

Section 2: Strategies to Prevent Care-refusal Behavior

Appearance and Overall Approach

During a recent home visit, one of my nieces took my picture without my knowledge. I was listening intently to something my sister was telling me. The picture surprised me. I looked so serious and somewhat… mean. I was frowning and wrinkling up my forehead. I had no idea I looked like that. This made me think: when I'm working with people living with dementia, do I look like this when I'm focused?

Gently smile. Relax your forehead. These two small steps will soften your features and make you appear more relaxed and friendly. People living with dementia, especially in the moderate to severe stages, rely more on non-verbal cues than spoken language.

Use Gentle Touch

This strategy is definitely person-dependent. Some people readily accept having their hands gently held and their back gently rubbed. Touch is a powerful communication tool. Touch can be reassuring, like a hug. If you are unsure how the person living with dementia will respond to touch, start with the hands. If the person clasps your hands and smiles, you can try gently rubbing their should and upper back.

Short 1-step Commands

As the dementia gets worse, people with the disease have trouble keeping up with long sentences or explanations. Remember the shrinking box and messy closet? You will have more success with using short, one-step respectful commands/requests or, in some cases, more gestures and pantomime and fewer words. While you are using gestures and pantomime, try to keep smiling and a calm manner. In some cases, if you are doing the activity with your family member, like brushing your hair or eating, you are giving helpful cues to the person with dementia.

Gestures and Pantomime

Support what you want to say with gestures and pantomime, as if you are playing charades. I will make a "come with me" gesture with my hands. I also NEVER hold or pull someone with dementia. The result is a tug-of-war, and you will lose. Instead, I gently place their hands on my wrists and I walk backwards or side-by-side. Try it. Also, nod your head and smile when you are getting the response you want.

Make it Vague

Instead of saying, "Let's go brush your teeth," try "Let's go have fun." Don't judge, I know it sounds super weird (and creepy). For reasons I have not yet figured out, I have gotten people to the bathroom with the fun sentence.

Encourage self-care...no matter how long it takes!

One of the best ways to prevent care refusals and resistance is to encourage the person with dementia to perform as much of his or her own care as is safely possible. This is good for several reasons. First, if you start taking over and "doing for" your family member, the person may forget how to do that activity. Once the activity is forgotten, that memory may be gone for good. On the other hand, if you encourage the person with dementia to remain active and perform as much self-care and other activities as possible, you keep the memories "alive." Another reason is to provide a sense of accomplishment. When I complete a task, I usually feel good. The same goes for people living with dementia. **The desire to be useful and to have a purpose does not go away, but the outlets for this drive and desire diminish as the dementia gets worse.** Also, some of these activities can help the person with dementia reminisce and relive positive memories.

Schedules and Routines

Schedules and routines go hand-in-hand with self-care. Think about your own schedules and routines. I have a very specific morning routine and if it gets messed up, like if I forget to set my alarm and wake up late, the rest of the day seems to go downhill. I will forget to bring the lunch I packed, or worse, walk out the door without my cell phone. My schedule serves as a type of reminder so that I head to work with everything I need for the day.

Schedules and routines also help to support memory and function in persons with dementia. Familiar schedules and routines are comforting in a world where things can be confusing. You can also use schedules and routines to help prevent care refusals. One family I knew was having trouble getting mom to take a bath. They began giving her a bath in the evening and entered her reality (more on that in later in the chapter) by telling her that everyone was bathing "before church tomorrow."

If your family member needs your help with some activity, your overall approach sets the tone. Make sure you have given yourself and your loved one enough time to complete the activity. Come at or below eye level in an unhurried way. Smile. It also helps to have the area set up for whatever activity you plan to do, like in the picture that follows. Notice that the toothbrush and other supplies are out and ready to go.

Avoid Elderspeak (baby talk)

Sometimes, the person with dementia may act in a child-like manner. Whatever you do, never talk to the person like he or she is a child. The person with dementia may forget a great deal about him or herself, but these folks will never forget that they are adults. Some caregivers forget themselves and start to use sing-song baby talk. This type of speech is called "elderspeak" and it will make refusals worse.

Use the Environment to Trigger Memories

In Chapter 5, I talked about memories becoming lost and mixed up using the shrinking box and messy closet examples. Memories are lost in the reverse order in which they are made. You can use the environment to "pull up" a deep memory. This is called **"priming**." For instance, some caregivers try to be efficient and attempt to brush their loved ones' teeth in the shower or while the person is sitting on the toilet. Instead, use the environment in a way that makes sense. If you are trying to get your family member to brush his or teeth, for example, help him or her to sit/stand in front of the sink and start the water running.

Ask for Help

All of us want to be needed and to have a job or purpose. Let's say your loved one refuses to eat, and you know they didn't eat much dinner last night. You know they need to get something in their stomach. You could "ask for help" by saying, "I made extra. Don't want the food to be wasted. Can you help me?"

Chaining

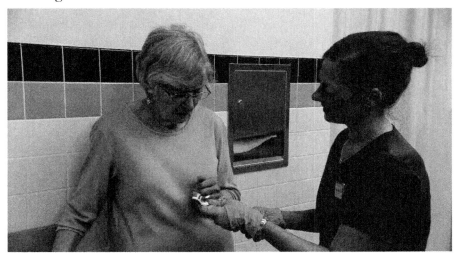

Chaining is starting the activity and having the person with dementia finish the activity. Click here to see the chaining video.

Watch your "Vibes"

Ever hear of "emotional contagion?" It is the spread of some emotion from one person to another. Yes, just like spreading a cold. There are people who brighten a room just be walking into it. There are others who also brighten up a room... as they go out the door! The human body has nerves whose only job is to "pick up" and send vibrations to the brain. So when someone says, "I don't get a good vibe about that person," this is not woohooey new age stuff but legit nerve activity.

After a rough day at work and heading to your "second shift," or after hearing "Where have you been?" for the 10 millionth time (and you have been RIGHT FREAKING HERE!!!) it can be a little hard to be chill and keep one's vibes "in check." So, go ahead. Scream. Preferably outside or in a pillow or some where not likely to result in a phone call to the cops. Personally, I find swearing very therapeutic (not at my loved one!). I go to another room and allow a couple of minutes of St.-George-Carlin-would-be-proud language. Or I call my sister and just go into a profanity-laden tirade which doesn't hurt anyone (except embarrass her because she foolishly had me on speakerphone as she was walking through a crowded hospital corridor... she just shrugged and told everyone that I had Tourette's.) If that doesn't do it, I walk out to my yard and hug an old magnolia tree (after dodging the spiderwebs). Again, I realize that sounds fruit loops but it works for me.

Once I fix my vibes, I'm ready to go back and face the situation. This time out usually results in my loved one having a break (and hopefully forgetting that I was being a butt).

Moving Backwards in Time/Entering Their Reality

Sometimes people living with dementia literally move backwards in time. Also, time starts to lose its structure. Your family member may tell you, "I've already had breakfast." Instead of arguing with your family member, or using logic by pointing to the time on the clock, simply go along with it. One way to respond is to say, "Oh, OK. I'm going to make myself some toast because I'm still hungry." Then, make the breakfast and serve it to your family member. If your loved one persists with, "I already ate," you can respond with, "OK, I made some extra and I don't want it to go to waste."

When I began my nursing career in the mid-1980s, we were taught to "present reality" to persons living with dementia. I found out the hard way that this approach was terrible. I was working the night shift. At 2 a.m., one of the residents awoke and climbed out of bed because she "had to catch a train to get to work." I did was I was being taught to do in nursing school. I escorted her back to her bed, helped her climb in, and calmly explained that she was at Saint Joseph's Nursing Home and it was 1984. It was 2 am and she needed to go back to sleep. Guess what happened? She climbed out of bed again. This futile activity went on for a good eternity (ok, 5 minutes). Each time that I "presented reality," the resident became more anxious and resisted returning to bed. Another nursing assistant walked into the room. She took the resident's hand, smiled, and calmly said, "It's OK. The train doesn't leave until 8 am. I'll wake you up at 6 am and make sure you have a good breakfast, and then you can catch the train with the other girls." The lady rolled over and went to sleep. The nursing assistant looked at me like I was a moron because I was a nursing student and should have known better.

At 2:30 am in 1984 at Saint Joseph's Manor, I learned that "presenting reality" was utter bullshit. Instead, I had just been introduced to "Therapeutic Fibbing."

Should I Lie to Get Them to Cooperate? Introducing "Therapeutic Fibbing"

In 1999, two social workers by the names of Beach and Kramer coined the term "therapeutic fibbing." They described "therapeutic fibbing" as a quick way to derail behavior that is distressing to the person with dementia or the caregiver. Usually the caregiver. In the above experience, the nursing assistant engaged in therapeutic fibbing. I became a fan. I used therapeutic fibbing in a variety of situations. I even documented "therapeutic fibbing" in my charts as an acceptable strategy.

Fast forward to 2011. I was running a large research study where we were testing ways to provide mouth care to people living with dementia in nursing homes. I was helping one of the residents living in the Memory Care Unit brush her teeth. She was asking about her mother. Automatically, I responded that her mother would be back "later, because she was at the store." The resident suddenly stopped brushing her teeth and abruptly said, "My mother died years ago." She then fixed me with a hateful stare. My stomach just dropped.

The next day, I hoped that I would be operating from a clean slate. Sort of. Everything started out smoothly but then she became very resistant towards my mouth care attempts. I excused myself and had another person approach her. No problems. Every time I approached, the nursing home resident became visibly upset and agitated.

From Therapeutic Fibbing to Entering Their Reality

My last experience with therapeutic fibbing caused me to rethink this approach. I now believe that our vibes can alter when we engage in therapeutic fibbing. After all, I know that people's voices and vital signs can change when they are being deceitful. I also realized the danger with therapeutic fibbing. One never knows which memory will become accessible—which happened with the resident I described in the above section. I've had people living with dementia not recognize their spouse one moment, then suddenly make the connection a few moments later. I suspect that I may make things worse if I am "caught" in a lie because a certain memory happens to surface just as the wrong words spill out of my mouth.

I also wondered if therapeutic fibbing was a handy shortcut that robbed us of the chance to explore emotions and unmet needs underlying the pleas to "find my mom" or "go home." Does "where is my mother" really mean "I don't feel safe"? No matter how old I become, or how frail she becomes, my mother is linked to feelings of safety, of being loved, and of being cared for. Every time something serious happens, who do I call? Mom. It would make sense, then, that if I become very forgetful, I would be looking for, and asking for, my mother.

"Entering their reality" is a strategy that helps us to communicate with the person living with dementia. It has two sides to it. On one side, when someone is asking to go home or looking for a long-lost relative, we reminisce: "What do you like most about xx?" "What favorite food did your grandmother make?" If we are faced with care refusals, such as "I just brushed my teeth" when it is very obvious that the teeth have not been brushed for some time, we enter their reality and produce a reason that makes sense in their world.

When you think about it, we enter everyone's reality all of the time. It is a way to provide feedback that is helpful, affirming, and kind. **Think of "Entering Their Reality" as a gentle and kind approach to delivering truth with dignity.** Let's say I go shopping with my daughter, Sara. I select a dress with a tag that proclaims it to be a size 12 but, once on, fits more like a size 6. Sara has a choice. She can say:

- "Mom, you are way too fat for that dress."
- "Mom, that dress is not a good match for your body shape. It hides your best features."
- "Mom, I think somebody messed up and put the wrong tag on that dress. I think it may be cut way too small."

I like #2 or #3. All give the same message, "You do NOT look good in that dress." All contain ELEMENTS OF THE TRUTH. But the second and third options allow me to accept the situation (the dress does not fit me) but still feel good.

Entering Their Reality to Avoid Care-Refusals: Case Study

When I was teaching clinical in a local nursing home, there was a resident who was a retired attorney. He had early-onset Alzheimer's, which meant he was much younger than the other residents—and much stronger! He refused to allow the nursing assistants to remove his soiled clothing (he was incontinent of urine and feces) or to shower him. Two male nursing assistants would literally carry him into the shower and strip off his soiled clothing. It was a bad situation. Talk about triggering a fear response!! This forceful behavior escalated his refusals and left him upset and agitated for hours.

Loving a challenge, I decided to work with him. I tried all of the strategies listed in this chapter with partial success. I could get him into the bathroom and could remove some clothing, but then he would have NONE OF IT and would walk out. One morning, I was accompanied by a nursing student who came from a family of attorneys. Before I could say a word, she jumped in. She looked at him and said, "The judge is waiting. Let's get you ready."

Holy shit!! The resident jumped out of his chair and my nursing student took him by the hand and led him to the bathroom. Using gestures, pantomimes, and very simple one-step commands, she single-handedly undressed and showered him. Whenever he would start to resist, she would simply repeat, "The judge is waiting in chambers. Let's get you ready." Success!

After she was finished with his care, I asked about her approach. She told me that her grandfather, who was the same age as this individual, told her stories of putting in long hours working on a case, sometimes pulling all-nighters. This was also a time when attorneys often kept alcohol in their office and would sometimes have a few drinks before leaving the office. Her grandfather always kept a fresh shirt and toiletries in the office. This way, if he received a message that he was expected in a judge's chambers, he could quickly freshen up so that he didn't look like he had been working (or drinking) all night. It was considered bad form to show up in the judge's chambers looking like hell.

"I simply used your 'entering his reality' approach, Dr. Jablonski. Somewhere, there are judges sitting in their chambers. Maybe they are waiting for their lunch. Maybe they are waiting for a meeting. I put two sentences together that I suspected would make him want to get cleaned up. I tapped into his old memories, like you are always talking about."

DAMN!! This was one of the high points of my teaching career!!

When faced with care refusals, think about your family member's past life and values. You may be able to come up with a "reason" to do something that is not lying and is something that is important to them. I will go into more ways to apply "Entering Their Reality" when I do a deep dive into bathing, mouth care, and medications—common activities that trigger care-refusal behavior.

How Denial Can Cause Care-Refusals (and what to do about it!)

There is a term called **"anosognosia"** (pronounced ah-no-so-NO-see-ya), which means persons living with dementia are completely unaware of their memory problems. **This is different from denial.** Here is how denial is different from anosognosia. When I am in denial about something, I <u>choose</u> to ignore a scary problem or to see the scary problem as "not so bad" so that I can temporarily deal with life. Denial is a defense mechanism. When I am finally mentally able to handle the situation, my denial breaks. This is because deep down in my brain, I **knew** that I was facing a scary problem. I had to mentally "bury" the scary problem until I was able to face it. Believe it or not, denial can be a healthy TEMPORARY coping method. People get in trouble when denial becomes a way of life, but that is another topic for another day!

Anosognosia, on the other hand, **happens because I forget that I forgot.** If I am unable to remember that I have a scary problem, then I simply do not have a scary problem. **I forgot that I just asked you the same question 5 times. I forgot that I nearly wrecked the car. I forgot that I got lost coming home from the store yesterday.** Now, when you tell me that this is the 6th time I'm asking the same question, *I become angry because NO IT IS NOT! I'VE NEVER ASKED YOU THAT QUESTION. THIS IS THE FIRST TIME I ASKED IT!* Or, if you tell me that I got lost yesterday coming home from the store, *I'm going to look at you like you are crazy because I don't remember getting lost yesterday. What the hell are YOU talking about???*

Self-Awareness

Some people living with dementia, usually vascular dementia or primary progressive aphasia (another type of FTD), maintain some self-awareness and realize that they have memory problems. These people may become sad and depressed because they can feel their memories or abilities slipping away. However, for many who have Alzheimer's dementia, they lose that self-awareness as it pertains to their memory problems. **Without that self-awareness, because of "forgetting that I forgot," reminders and "education" is not a good idea.**

Using "Entering Their Reality" When Dealing with Anosognosia

Now that I've explained the difference between anosognosia and denial, I'm going to have to say that constantly telling someone he or she has dementia may be worthless—and may instead trigger a lot of arguments and unpleasantness. People living with dementia at the moderate stage may suddenly decide they do not need a "dementia pill" like Donepezil because "they don't have dementia." I find a non-dementia reason and help the family member with a script such as, "you have diabetes and high blood pressure, both diseases can hurt your memory. This pill can help your memory stay as healthy as possible." Yes, it is a stretch, but this approach is grounded in truth.

Putting It All Together

At first, some of these ideas will feel weird. Play with the techniques, and see what works best for you and your family member. I have some patients with whom I barely speak because the spoken words trigger unwelcome or difficult (for me) behaviors. I have other patients with whom I sing the entire time I'm providing care. It is somewhat trial and error, but the results are worth the experimentation!

Section 3: Dealing with Refusals in Real-Time

You are in the middle of bathing your mom and she starts trying to leave the tub. Or, you cannot even get your father into the shower. In this section, I will describe ways to handle care-resistant behavior in the moment. There is some repetition between this section and the earlier section of Chapter 7; that is because some techniques are handy for both preventing care refusals and managing care refusals in the moment. It is important to pay attention to what was going on RIGHT before the behavior happened, because the timing may provide clues for WHY your family member started to resist or refuse the care.

Enter Their Reality ("Dementia Land")

Entering their reality is a good way to prevent care refusals, but it can also be used to handle care refusals. You may have to approach the activity in a way that makes sense to their past memories and experiences. For example, one woman would agree to being showered but became hysterical when her daughter tried to wash her hair. The daughter tried washing her mother's hair last, but then her mother started trying to get out of the shower halfway through. After the daughter and I spoke, we both realized that her mother used to have her hair washed and styled weekly. The daughter, in fact, began recalling humorous situations where her mother took great lengths to prevent her hair from getting wet in-between hair styling appointments. The daughter decided to give mom a shower but used a shower cap. Mom stopped fighting the showers.

Distraction

Distraction is another useful technique. One can try singing familiar songs or asking the family member to talk about a favorite memory. We have found that singing is a very powerful distraction, but it works best if you know your family member's musical preferences or favorite songs.

Bridging

Bridging involves using an object related to the care activity at hand. In this video clip, https://www.youtube.com/watch?v=tP0I4IH9fu8 we used a toothbrush as a bridging object. Bridging is similar to priming. You are trying to use familiar objects to access the memories around the activity you are trying to do.

Hand-over-Hand

Sometimes, you can help reduce care-resistant behavior by using a hand-over-hand technique. There are a couple of ways to do this. The first is to place your hands over that of the person with dementia, and guide their hands with yours. Another way is to place their hands over yours, and continue with the care.

Mirror-Mirror

Mirror-mirror works best with mouth care, but it can also work well for dressing. Helping the person in front of a mirror is similar to using the environment to support memories of self-care. Sometimes, though, performing mouth care serves as a type of distraction...especially if the person with

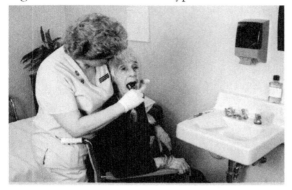

dementia does not recognize him or herself in the mirror. If the person with dementia becomes upset and thinks the mirror images are strangers watching him or her, do not use this technique.

Caregiver Vibes

Sometimes, persons with dementia may refuse care because they are feeling rushed or may have forgotten, halfway through the activity, that they were in the middle of toileting, bathing, or getting dressed. When you start to encounter refusals, first check your own feelings. Are you starting to feel anxious or rushed? Upset? If so, take a deep breath and tell yourself, "I'm doing fine." Because, you really are.

Ask for Help

Next, try asking for help, using short, one-step requests. For example, saying "Can you help me with this shirt?" while gesturing that you want your father to put his arm in the sleeve.

Apologize with Praise

Also, if the person seems to be getting upset, apologize. An apology with praise can also short-circuit care-resistant behavior: "I am sorry, I don't feel like I'm doing this right. You are so patient with me." Think about it. How many times in a day does someone apologize to you AND give you a compliment? Probably not much.

Rewards

If none of these seem to be helping, you may want to bring up some positive type of reward. "Once we are finished, we are going to have some ice cream." Or, "after this, we can see the grandkids."

Rescue

As an absolutely last resort, and if you have another family member nearby, you can use the "rescue" approach. If the care refusals are escalating, and this is something that absolutely needs to happen (like changing soiled underwear), have the other family member step in and tell you to leave. Then, have the new person remove the soiled clothes. Rescue needs to be used carefully—you want person #2 to be someone liked by the person with dementia.

***

I have an awesome free resource—a guide with all of these tips that you can print out and keep handy. Go to https://dementiacentricsolutions.com/caring-for-someone-living-with-dementia-tired-of-fighting-and-arguing/ and get your free guide today!

CHAPTER 10

Bathing, Mouth Care, and Care Refusals

In Chapter 9, I provided general strategies for preventing and managing care-refusal behavior. In this chapter, I will describe how to apply some of the strategies to refusals around mouth care and bathing.

Bathing and Care Refusals

Many family caregivers encounter issues with bathing. The first issue is frequency. Many older adults came from a time period where they sponged off most days and had a full immersed bath once or twice a week. Also, frequent bathing can dry out older skin and cause itching. Unless there is an incontinence problem, if bathing is a battle it may be better to wash at the sink and invoke the reality of the "Saturday night bath."

Do not ask, "Do you want to shower or bathe?" Otherwise, you will get the "automatic no" and it is hard to recover after that. Instead, using some of the techniques in chapter 9 . One of my favorite techniques for getting someone into the bathroom is to have them hold my wrists while I walk backward into the bathroom. Just make sure you have a clear path and you know your bathroom layout.

Use the environment to trigger memories. Bathe the person in the tub or shower (if safely possible). Make sure the bathroom is warm and not drafty. Have all of the supplies and towels in reach. Have the person with dementia perform as much of the washing as she or he can. Some couples shower together. I've even had some daughters shower with mom and sons with dads. Do whatever works. Some of my families have had good success with turning the shower/bath into a "spa" experience, especially with women. They use scented candles, extra fluffy towels, music, and special soaps. Just make sure if you go this route, you don't create a fire or fall hazard with slippery oils.

For situations where your family member needs more help, a shower chair or bar may be necessary to prevent falls. Start by spraying the feet and working up towards the neck. Save washing the hair for last, or save hair washing for the hair salon. It may be helpful to let the person hold and control the shower wand; this is an example where hand-over-hand may prevent the water from going all over the place but allow the person with dementia to feel in control.

Sometimes, covering the person with towels and removing a towel at a time, washing that body part, then putting the towel back, may reduce care resistance for 2 reasons: modesty and warmth. I've given many showers in my time and while I may be sweating profusely, the person I was showering was shivering. Another technique that works is using a terry cloth bathing suit coverup and placing it backwards, so that it is open in the back. This way, you can wash their back and butt and legs, then turn the robe around so that it is open in the front and finish the bath/shower.

As mentioned in previous sections of this book, allow the person with dementia to complete as much of the bath/shower as possible. For people living with dementia who do not want help, you may want to offer to "wash your back" or "help with the feet." Think about it. I would feel OK about someone helping me to wash my back or wash my feet, and I would accept that help. No way would I want someone trying to wash more intimate areas, that would freak me out!! If your loved one needs that level of help, and they are refusing it, you can use the hand-over-hand technique mentioned in Chapter 9.

Mouth Care

People living with dementia may refuse mouth care for a couple of reasons. Is the electric/battery toothbrush something they learned to use after age 50? If so, they may have lost the memory of an electric toothbrush but may tolerate a manual one. Are they experiencing mouth pain? Until you can get them to a dentist, gently brush over that area with a soft, manual toothbrush.

Proximal brushes or interdentate sticks are better than flossing. Speak to your dentist about products that will work best for your family member. In my research study, where we provided mouth care to people living with dementia who resisted care, we used plastic interdentate sticks. We asked our participants to "pick their teeth with the toothpick." It worked! We also used gestures, pantomimes, chaining, bridging, and distraction to complete mouth care.

***

I have an awesome free resource—a guide with all of these tips that you can print out and keep handy. Go to https://dementiacentricsolutions.com/caring-for-someone-living-with-dementia-tired-of-fighting-and-arguing/ and get your free guide today!

CHAPTER 11

Dressing and Care Refusals

This chapter builds on information covered in Chapter 9. In this chapter, I will explain how to tailor these general approaches to care refusals around dressing.

"Let's Get Dressed" NOT "Do you want to get dressed?

It may be best to introduce the topic of dressing as a stated activity, not as a question. Allow the older adult to dress as independently as possible. As dementia gets worse, it becomes more difficult to select outfits or remember the order in which the clothes should be put on. You can help by laying the clothes out in order or handing them to your family member one at a time. Use prompts, either in the form of short, 1-step requests or by gesturing and pantomiming. If someone is really resistant to getting dressed, it can be helpful to use the "ask for help" technique by asking them to show you how to put on an item of clothing.

Avoid Rushing

Avoid rushing the person living with dementia. Your "vibe" changes when you are in a hurry. If you are feeling impatient, you may cause the person living with dementia to feel upset. Upset feelings often lead to care refusals.

Keep It Simple

Sometimes, we provide too much information. True, adults want to know why they have to do something. It needs to make sense to us. Persons living with dementia may have mixed up and fragmented memories. They may also have problems following a line of reasoning. For example:

"Mom, please get dressed. You are going to the doctor."

"Why do I need to go to the doctor? I'm fine."

See where this is going? Now, you are getting into a "hamster wheel" of futile discussion about the doctor's visit. Instead, shift gears and simplify the situation.

"Mom, it is time to get dressed."

"Why? I'm fine."

"I know. But it is time to get dressed. This mango shirt looks great on you! It is one of my favorites."

It may feel weird, but sometimes simply repeating a very simple fact is all that is needed.

Entering Their Reality

If you are getting refusals, try to think about possible situations from their past that may help trigger memories of getting dressed. For example, what daily routine did the person living with dementia follow? Were they awakened every morning by an alarm? Was the routine getting dressed and then eating breakfast? Sometimes dressing refusals happen because we have changed up the routine due to our needs. We teach children routines to help them make memories. For people living with dementia, we keep routines to help keep the memories.

Literal Placement

I lay out my clothes on my bed prior to putting them on. My pants are zipper side up; I flip them around to step into them. If I had moderate dementia, I would not recall this step. Instead, I would pick up the pants (with the zipper facing me) and put them on backward.

If this is something you are noticing, simply lay the clothes out so that the person living with dementia can put them on without turning the item around. This means placing the pants zipper side down on the bed.

Bottom Line

It is best to have the person living with dementia do as much dressing as is safely possible. Sometimes it is tempting to dress the person to save time. Here is the issue: every time a person living with dementia performs an activity, the neurons involved in that activity are exercised. The nerves are used. If you dress the person, you stop the nerves involved in the activity from being used. Over time, the nerves will shrivel up. The person living with dementia may not have enough extra nerves to pick up the activity. The ability is lost forever. I go deeper into this information in Chapter 12.

***

I have an awesome free resource—a guide with all of these tips that you can print out and keep handy. Go to https://dementiacentricsolutions.com/caring-for-someone-living-with-dementia-tired-of-fighting-and-arguing/ and get your free guide today!

Medication Refusals

"I don't need to take that medication. There is nothing wrong with me."
Sound familiar?

Are the Medications *ABSOLUTELY* Necessary?

At least once a week I'm on the phone with a family caregiver dealing with this issue. One of the first things I talk about is which meds we can safely stop. Did you know that proton-pump inhibitors, such as Prilosec(TM) (omeprazole) are for short-term use (a couple of weeks, maybe a month or two) only? And that the rebound symptoms of really bad heartburn can be minimized by titrating (weaning down) the dosage? So yes, the first thing I do is work with the family member and strongly encourage him or her to speak with the primary care provider about reducing the number of medications. If the PCP is part of the larger health care system where I practice, I contact the clinician directly.

Entering THEIR Reality

Persons with dementia may forget that they have health issues that require medication. Sometimes, taking medication together may help normalize the experience. You may also need to repeat the short, simple explanations, and enter their reality. By "entering their reality," you come up with reasons THAT MAKES SENSE to the person with dementia and REFLECTS HIS OR HER VALUES.

One of my patients, who had a heart attack as a young man, will take any pill if his wife tells him it is for his heart. THIS MAKES SENSE TO HIM. He has forgotten many things, but not that he had a heart attack.

One of my ladies told her husband that his pills were all various types of Viagra—I'm not sure I'd recommend that, because it may have another consequence. In this particular case, taking a pill that could enhance his performance MADE SENSE to this particular individual.

My personal favorite, because this reason would work with me, was provided by an adult caregiver: "Mom, these pills will help you to look younger." Mom always took pride in her appearance, and she was a beautiful woman, so her daughter tapped into mom's VALUE SYSTEM. And daughter was somewhat correct: if mom took her medication and felt better, she would look better, too. Maybe even younger.

Swallowing Problems

As dementia gets worse, some people begin to have problems with swallowing pills and will chew them. This is an example of forgetting how to do things in the reverse order of how they were learned. Children start with chewable vitamins, then progress to swallowing pills later. If swallowing a pill is the issue, talk to your provider about switching medications to liquid, chewable, or patch alternatives.

CHAPTER 13

How to Make These Strategies Your Own

The bulk of this book contains information about specific strategies for preventing and handling many dementia-driven behaviors. In order to figure out which strategies are best for a person, and in order to tweak the strategies so that they are personalized—which means they work for YOUR loved one, I use the following approach:

> **BRAIN SHRINKAGE (NEURODEGENERATION) + PERSONALITY**
> **+ VALUES + COHORT = BEHAVIORS**

Brain Shrinkage

If a person has a lot of shrinking in the frontal lobes but the hippocampi are healthy, that person will have problems with appropriate social behavior and judgement BUT will be able to score high on many of the memory tests that are used in clinics. This is what you see with people who have FTD. On the other hand, a person with Alzheimer's dementia has shrinking of the hippocampi while the frontal lobes remain healthy (at least in the beginning of the disease). This person will ask the same question multiple times and perform poorly on the typical memory tests used in clinics, but will behave appropriately in social situations. I had the experience of working with a person who had severe Alzheimer's dementia and who belched while I was feeding her breakfast. Even though she rarely spoke, she looked right at me and quietly said, "Excuse me."

Different patterns of brain shrinkage—of neurodegeneration—guide strategy choices. The person with FTD with shrinkage in the frontal and temporal lobes who just wants to sit on the couch and veg—because of the apathy that comes with FTD—may respond best to the chaining strategy. This is where you start the action, like getting dressed, and have the person with FTD finish the action. When you use chaining, you are compensating for the shrinking parts of the brain that are having a lot of trouble with starting any action. For a person with AD, I would recommend cueing. Cueing is breaking down an activity, like dressing, into multiple steps and reminding the person with dementia what step to take: "Put your arm in the sleeve. Pull the sleeve up. Put your other arm in the sleeve. Button the top button. Button the next." Cueing may annoy a person with FTD who still has much more short-term memory than a person with AD.

Personality

A person's pre-disease personality is another important piece of the dementia behavior puzzle. Before the dementia, was the person a social butterfly, planning social events and always on the move? Was the person a reader who preferred quiet indoor activities to hiking or camping? How did the person cope with problems? Did they talk it out or walk it out? Personality can shine a light on many behaviors that are a way of coping with the brain changes that occur with the dementias.

Someone who was always physically active their entire life may default to physical movement when they feel upset or confused. Family caregivers may try to restrict movement in order to keep the person living with dementia "safe." On the contrary, the well-meaning family members are making the need to move even worse! Some families make sure the outside yard is secure and the fence is locked, giving the person living with dementia a safe space to move. Others make sure that doors leading to the outside have alarms and locks that are out of reach for the person living with dementia.

When I first started working with family caregivers, I encountered a very frustrated spouse whose wife was diagnosed with FTD. He followed her around the house and constantly attempted to have her "help" with household chores. She became increasingly angry and at one point, started throwing cleaning supplies in his direction. After some careful questioning, I learned that the two of them ran the family business: she handled the administrative activities while he spent a great deal of time "on the road" with clients. He sold the business and retired when his wife was diagnosed with the FTD. Now I realized the problem. She was accustomed to doing her own thing and did not like being "micromanaged" by her spouse. She also despised cleaning; she always hired a cleaning person so that she could do the administrative activities that she enjoyed! Together, we came up with a strategy in which she could have her own desk with an adding machine, pencil sharpeners, legal pads, and other office supplies. When he had to hire a part-time caregiver, his wife was elated—she thought he had hired her a secretary! By aligning the strategies with his wife's personality (and her preferences), he avoided the anger and rage and had a much better relationship with his wife.

Values

My father was a bit of a rogue and had several extra-marital affairs. Because of this experience, I was overly concerned about marrying someone who would be unfaithful. I was so completely focused on finding a spouse who would be faithful that I failed to notice other traits that ultimately resulted in a very unhappy marriage and subsequent divorce. I learned an extremely hard lesson!

Let's imagine that I had decided to stay in the marriage. Fast forward 40 or 50 years, and I have developed dementia. As I move backwards in time, my fear of infidelity may bubble back up to the surface. I begin to show delusions—false beliefs—that my spouse is being unfaithful. Perhaps this delusion is also being triggered by his lack of interaction with me because he is completely overwhelmed by the caregiving role. Delusions are very difficult to derail, but often just realizing where the delusions may be coming from is helpful.

Values can also help with tailoring a strategy. Parents value helping their children. One strategy that works very well when used by adult children caring for their parents with dementia is "asking for help." "Mom, can you help me by putting on this shirt?"

Cohort

Knowing the time period when persons living with dementia were teens and young adults is also very helpful in understanding behaviors and tailoring approaches. I recall my experiences as a nursing assistant in the early 1980s. Many of the nursing home residents with dementia had been born at the turn of the century. Some of the ladies in my care wore elaborate brassieres, girdles, garter belts, and thigh-high stockings. Even those with moderate dementia insisted on wearing these very challenging undergarments. After one frustrating morning of trying to help one of the residents with the bra/girdle combination from hell, I thought to myself: "Should I become a nursing home resident, I wonder if I will be insisting on wearing my tight bootcut jeans and push-up bras?"

The use of "gadgets" is very different, depending on cohort. My cohort is Gen X. I learned how to use a "desktop" computer in my late 20s and became proficient in software that no longer exists, like Wordperfect™. I had dial-up internet which I thought was the coolest thing ever because I could read email and "surf the web" at 2 am while breastfeeding my daughter. Now I get pissed off if I'm looking for research articles and they are not available digitally…but I still print them out to read them because I like highlighting important points and writing notes in the margin. Contrast my experience with the Gen Z cohort (born after 1998). The Gen Z cohort grew up with more access to electronics (smartphones, tablets, and laptops) and earlier exposure to these devices than Gen X. In chapter 1, I described the loss of abilities as moving backward in time, where people lose their ability to correctly use items and appliances in the reverse order they learned them. This means that a person from Gen X with dementia will lose the ability to use smartphones and computers earlier in the disease than a person from Gen Z, because the Gen X person learned to use these device later in life. Conversely, clinicians in the future who are treating Gen Z-ers with dementia will notice that the ability to use computers and smart phones are retained later in the disease.

Language and acceptable social behaviors are based in one's cohort. Socially acceptable language changes depending on the time period. For example, "acceptable" profanity in the media has evolved. In the 1970s, one would rarely hear anything stronger than "damn." Words like "ass" and "bitch" can be heard even on network shows now. Terms around race, ethnicity, and gender identity also continue to evolve. This is why people living with dementia may use racial or ethnic terms that make us cringe today but were part of the "acceptable" language in the 1960s.

Dementia Behavior Coaching May Be the Answer!

Learning all of this information may be very overwhelming! It may be easier to sign up for one of my dementia behavior courses. This way, you have access to me. I can help you identify the best strategies for difficult behaviors and help you personalize the strategies so that they make sense for your family member!

Dementia behavior coaching or signing up for a dementia behavior course is no different than working with a personal trainer, taking a yoga class, or hiring someone to teach you how to play a musical instrument! Dementia behavior coaching or a dementia behavior course will save you time, energy, and a lot of aggravation and frustration! Check out the options on my course site, https://dementiacentricsolutions.com.

CHAPTER 14

Meaningful Interactions Support Function: Lessons Learned from Tony Bennett, Salmon Patties, and Fridge Worms

Interactions that Maximize Abilities: The Power of Procedural Memory

At the time of this writing, Tony Bennett gave a concert with Lady Gaga. In spite of severe memory loss, Mr. Bennett gave a flawless performance. This is an example of procedural memory. In Mr. Bennett's case, he had sung his songs thousands of times over decades. His "library of songs" is an over-learned skill. For most of us, skills like reading are over-learned. We learn to read in pre-school or kindergarten and then read every day for the rest of our lives.

Every time we do a specific activity, we reinforce the neural network that is responsible for the activity. Think of it this way... It is morning and I walk my dog across my lawn. I turn around, and I see my footprints and Amira's dog prints in the wet grass. When we come back from our walk, our footprints are gone. The grass has sprung back into its original shape. This is what happens in the brain when we do something once and never do it again. Or only do it once a year or once every couple of years. The memory "path" is very faint or completely disappears. On the other hand, if we do something daily, or multiple times a day, we create literal "roads" in the brain that are made of layers of neurons. These roads are similar to the path in my yard where no grass grows. The previous owner, who lived here for 25 years, always had dogs. They ran around the yard along the fence. This constant dog traffic has created a dirt path. Now my dog runs around the same yard, reinforcing that dirt path. If we move tomorrow and the new owner does not have dogs, the dirt path may become grown over with grass and weeds. It will probably take a few years for the grass and other plants to completely erase the dirt path.

In the case of Tony Bennett, his wife encouraged him to sing daily, listen to his music, and look at photo albums to keep his memory roads clear and working. Her efforts helped him to maintain his access to all of his memories that helped him to perform at his concert.

Maintaining Function

Well-meaning family and formal caregivers sometimes start to "overdo" for persons living with dementia. "I don't want her to get hurt" or "I don't want him to feel embarrassed" or "It is just so much easier if I do (fill in the blank)." **What people do not realize is that once a person with dementia forgets how to do an activity or task, he or she is rarely able to relearn it. There just aren't enough nerve cells and brain chemicals to knit together a new memory.**

I (stupidly) remarried in 2014 and became the carer for my (now ex) husband's mother who had dementia. When I first met Mary, she was sitting in her bathrobe in a recliner. She had just lost her husband of 60-plus years. She was a frail, sad, birdlike woman. She needed a walker and could get to and from the bathroom. Her son was extremely concerned that she would fall and injure herself, so he constantly told her to sit down. Like every 10 minutes. If he found her standing or walking around the house, he would fuss: "Go sit down before you hurt yourself." She was miserable.

When I became her caregiver, I encouraged her to move around our house. I wanted to find things that Mary would enjoy doing. At the time, my husband traveled extensively for his work and was gone for days at a time. Without his constant fussing, Mary was essentially free! One of the first things I started was weekly outings, starting with a shopping trip for an updated wardrobe. Because Mary had lost so much weight, everything she owned was several sizes too big. Mary was thrilled; she began getting dressed every morning and sporting her new outfits.

I discovered that Mary had been an avid and talented gardener. She would talk about her flowers and plants for hours. Inspiration struck. I put several plastic tubs on my back deck and we planted herbs and flowers in them. We went out every evening after dinner and watered or weeded the tubs. Then we would sit out on the deck and read together. Mary started washing dishes and helping with light housework. She gained weight, became stronger, and seemed much happier. She still had dementia, but having her on a schedule and keeping her active helped her to stay fairly independent with her own care. Her decline was slowed down.

Every time her son returned from his business trips, he would fuss at both of us because of Mary's mobility. "She is going to fall and break something." What he failed to realize was that his "care" was not only making her more unhappy and depressed, he was increasing her risk of falling because he was keeping her from walking around regularly. **He was stealing away her ability to do things. When a person with dementia stops doing a task, they risk forgetting how to do that activity. As the disease moves on, they are unable to remake those memories.** When I encouraged Mary to make her salmon patties or to help with the flowers, I was keeping her task memories alive. I was pushing away the day where she would become dependent on others for her care.

And speaking of salmon patties, Mary made them every Friday for as long as she lived with us. Sadly, she died from congestive heart failure eight months after I became her caregiver. I'm grateful for the experience because it humbled me and enhanced my ability to help family caregivers!

Mary showed me that meaningful activities are very important for people living with dementia. I learned to modify her favorite activities so that she could engage in pleasurable hobbies. Who cares if the flowers go into the vase upside down. I had a family member become upset because the person with dementia drew pictures on the pages of the adult coloring book instead of coloring the pictures. Who cares???

One way to support abilities is to "chain," which means you start the activity and they finish. For example, you could place the colored pencil in a person's hand and guide their hand to start coloring the picture. Release, and see if the person will continue the activity. It is like priming a pump. And it usually works!

The sad thing is, abilities that are not consistently used with be lost. Forever. Because of the changes in the brain from dementia, new memories may not be able to be created.

Finding Outlets for People Living with Dementia

People living with dementia are vibrant, wonderful people...who happen to have a little, or maybe a lot, of forgetfulness. Here's the thing... the drive, the search for meaning, the desire for affection, the desire to be HEARD... remain. What changes is that the OUTLETS for the expression of these important desires and drives get cut off by the dementia... regardless of the type. The loss of these outlets creates anger, frustration, irritability and other behaviors. Sensitive and meaningful interactions with others can reduce the isolation felt by people liing with dementia.

My son, Mark, is an avid fisherman. When he lived at home, he kept his bait (those big red night crawlers) in the garage fridge, which also happens to be where I keep overflow food and defrosting items.

WARNING: THIS NEXT PART IS REALLY GROSS!!

One Saturday, I opened the garage fridge to retrieve some ground meat I had put in to defrost. There were FRIGGING GINORMOUS NIGHT CRAWLERS EVERYWHERE!! I lost it. Stephen King couldn't make this stuff up. Apparently, they either were hungry or were seeking an escape route or both. They had squeezed out of the foam container by pushing the plastic lid up (or maybe Mark hadn't closed it tightly enough). Another fun fact: these fuckers can scrunch themselves up so that they appear to be an inch long, but can stretch out to *NEARLY A FOOT!!* I found this out because all had stretched out to their maximum capacity. Some were stretched out within the folds of the white accordion gasket that lines the edge of the refrigerator door; others had tunneled through the plastic wrap of the meat and were feasting away. A couple of outliers were channeling their inner Spider-man by hanging on the sides of the fridge. I kid you not, I think there were 20 of these damn things so I'm not sure if they had had a worm orgy, invited friends, or simply engaged in cellular division.

At the time, the fridge was relatively new and in great working order (other than needing to be dewormed), so tossing it out was not an option. After unleashing my volcanic temper and spewing language that could melt titanium, I handed Mark a bucket, rags, and some bleach and put him in charge of Operation Worm Cleanup. I felt bad after the initial eruption of Mount Rita, so I helped. Mother-son bonding time, yay. And then inspiration struck.

These worms are a great metaphor for dementia-related behaviors!!!

The night crawlers did not have a meeting and decide to freak out the red-headed human. They were being worms. Worms move around and eat stuff. **I created the situation** by allowing the hungry worms to be in the fridge in the first place and then placing food in their vicinity.

The person with dementia does not do things to tick off the caregiver. **The individual's personality and drive and need for a purpose remain.** Dementia keeps those pieces boxed inside the person. **The person with dementia wants an outlet for that drive and energy but is no longer able to channel these desires into appropriate (for us) venues.** If I do not provide an outlet for that energy, drive, or purpose, then I create a problematic situation. **If the environment is not a good fit for the person's personality, you will see behaviors that may not make sense, may be dangerous or may increase the effort of caregiving.**

The trick is to **provide outlets by providing safe activities that are aligned with the person's pre-dementia personality, occupation, and favorite hobbies.** That activity may have to be modified a bit to make it safe. For example, I have a neighbor with dementia who was an active gardener. He still loves to mow the lawn. Multiple times a day. No matter how hot outside, he is mowing the lawn. He will not stop until the mower runs out of gas. His wife was terrified of dehydration, heat stroke, or an injury from the mower. When his wife tried to bar him from mowing the lawn, he became extremely angry. So his wife gave up and let him mow the lawn to his heart's content.

Knowing what I do for a living, my neighbor's wife asked me for some ideas. I recommended a cordless electric lawn mower with the blades removed. I own two (that's another story for another day). I know from personal experience that you are lucky if the battery lasts an hour, even less on hot days. Their son took my advice and bought dad a new cordless electric mower for Father's Day. Son also removed the blades as an added precaution. Now, my neighbor mows for about an hour and the mower stops. He takes it into the garage, where his wife pulls out the battery and puts it on the charger. It takes a couple of hours for the battery to charge, creating a mandatory break. Win-win, everyone is happy.

And if you have nightcrawlers in your fridge, feed them cornmeal. If we had done that, they probably would have stayed in their container.

***

Want to learn more strategies? Subscribe to my newsletter, either with this URL or the QR code:

CHAPTER 15

Dementia and Living Life to the Fullest

Vacations, Travel, & Dementia

"I really want to travel or go on vacation with my family member who has dementia. What do you think?" My response is, "It depends on a couple of things."

Did the Person Living with Dementia Enjoy Traveling?

This may seem like a silly question, but it is really important. I personally love to BE in different places. I'm not a big fan of the PROCESS of getting there—especially if it involves air travel. My preference is train travel if the locale is accessible. What this means is if I should reach a point where I am diagnosed with some type of dementia, I would become apprehensive with travel activities.

Many times, we squelch our misgivings or dislikes because we know that the rewards from the final destination outweigh the hassle of getting there. When my children were young, I dreaded the annual family reunion in Sea Isle City, NJ. (Nothing against NJ beaches!) We lived in Richmond, Virginia. I had to coordinate ferry reservations, travel itineraries (for breast-feeding breaks/diaper changes/potty breaks—none of which EVER happened at the same time) and do 90% of the packing and meal planning. I did not breathe a sigh of relief until we pulled into the driveway of the beach house. And then, I had to coordinate the unpacking. My now-adult children have fond memories of these trips and were surprised to hear of my negative feelings about the actual trip.

If my kids were to put me in a car and take me to the beach somewhere, these old memories and anxieties may surface. I may become upset and want to "go home" or try to exit the car. My kids would be puzzled, "Mom always loved the ocean." Yup, Mom loves the ocean. She just hated the process of getting there.

Some friends of mine bought an RV and began traveling all over the US as soon as both retired. Twenty years ago. They love this adventure. One is starting to show signs of dementia. In this situation, the traveling piece is fine. She knows every inch of the RV. When they get to their destinations, however, she becomes anxious because the destinations seem unfamiliar.

Bottom Line

Honestly figure out if traveling, both the process of traveling and the end-result final destination, was pleasurable for the person living with dementia. If the answer to either is "no," stop. It would be better to stay-cation and invite friends and family to come to the person living with dementia.

How Severe is the Dementia?

The ability of the person to do self-care things is a good benchmark for dementia severity. People who can do everything but balance checkbooks, pay bills (correctly), and sensibly food shop are usually in the mild stage. Traveling and vacations should be OK, especially if the destination is somewhere familiar like the lake house or a relative's place.

Once the person living with dementia needs help with preparing meals and picking out the right clothes, he or she may be in the moderate stage. Here is where travel can get tricky. The person may wake up and forget where he or she is and try to leave. The person may fret and keep asking to go home, so the vacation is not really a vacation for the family member(s).

If the person living with vacation needs help going to the bathroom, it is likely that they are in the severe stage. Family restrooms are popping up all over airports. They are not the norm at rest stops. This is a challenge if the caregiver is one gender and the care-recipient is another. I had a male care-giver use the restroom himself, and his wife had wandered off in his very brief absence! This same caregiver is very creative. He learned that Publix grocery stores all have family restrooms. He planned his travel route based on access to Publix grocery stores and stopped there to access the family restrooms!

Bottom Line

The more severe the dementia, the less likely one should travel. Traveling takes a lot of mental energy. Persons with mild dementia have more mental energy than persons with severe dementia. This is why you may see more crankiness and irritability during travel as the dementia gets worse.

What is the Purpose of the Trip?

A better question is, "how important is it for the person living with dementia to be there?" Sometimes, WE want the person living with dementia to attend an event. Weddings, baptisms, bar mitzvahs—these are all happy and wonderful events. We want our family members to celebrate with us. I've had family members say, "This may be the last time everyone sees (insert name of person living with dementia)." Not true, these people can visit.

The decision to attend the event depends on the time of day, the size of the event, and the characteristics of the person living with dementia. A 100-person reception at 6 pm in the evening may stress out someone with even mild dementia. A brunch in a quiet restaurant with 10 people may be perfect for someone with moderate dementia.

Funerals are another issue. Spouses should have the opportunity to say good-bye. Again, this decision is informed by the severity of the dementia and (I hate to say this) the quality of the relationship. In one case, I suggested that the spouse with dementia attend the wake (near the end) and stay for the service as long as tolerated. This was after a long conversation with the adult children. In another case, the wife with dementia forgot she was even married, so attending the funeral of a spouse who had faded from memory seemed cruel.

I have also seen family caregivers appease other family members, even though the caregivers knew this was a bad idea. I often help family caregivers with "scripts" to deal with well-meaning but sometimes pushy relatives. We may say it different ways, but the bottom line is that the person living with dementia may not enjoy the event and may even become stressed by the event.

Bottom Line

The decision to attend an event is best made considering multiple factors. Ask the person living with dementia for their preferences. Weigh their expressed preferences with their pre-dementia personalities. Consider travel options, such as by car versus by plane. Determine if you can get assistance with both the travel process and with care once you get to the destination. Think about the size of the event, the number of people involved, and other logistics like timing.

Should you decide to embark on a vacation or travel activity, consider all of the ways things could go wrong and have a back-up plan. For example, I always travel with spare underwear in my computer bag in case my luggage goes AWOL. Have a travel bag with medications, wipes, and even a change of underwear in case a bathroom is not easily accessible. If traveling/staying at hotels, consider purchasing a cheap door alarm in case the person living with dementia makes an unplanned exit.

Good Resources

Dementia and Flying: https://www.dementia.org/how-to-fly-with-dementia

Is the Caregiver Equipped for Travel? https://dailycaring.com/6-ways-to-figure-out-if-traveling-with-dementia-will-work/

More Traveling Tips: https://alz.org/help-support/caregiving/safety/traveling

CHAPTER 16

Holidays & Dementia

Holidays are wonderful venues for celebrating important life events and visiting family members. Holidays are also stressful, even more so for dementia caregivers. This chapter discusses ways that dementia caregivers can adapt important holiday traditions and enjoy holidays with their loved ones.

Valentine's Day Message for Caregivers

Every year at the end of January/beginning of February, I post this message on my blog. It deserved to be part of this chapter. Enjoy!

Chocolates, plush animals, and romantic cards. Maybe even masks with cupid decorations. These are today's Valentine's Day staples. But want to see REAL LOVE in action? Watch a caregiver for someone with dementia.

(Apologies to Saint Paul; I used his First Letter to the Corinthians, verses 4-13, as the platform for this post).

Love really tries to be patient. Especially when I try to figure out why a certain behavior is happening. Love is kind; I play to his or her strengths instead of dwelling on the not-so-great parts.

Love gently provides the same answer to the same question asked 6 times in the last 5 minutes. Especially about the masks we have to wear now. Love sweetly listens to the same stories over and over again. Love is entering the person with dementia's reality to understand the behaviors.

Love is creative as I find meaningful activities that respect his or her preferences, which was even tougher when respite programs shut down and my loved one lost an important outlet. I was grateful for the weekly Zoom sing-a-longs, but it was just not the same.

Love is accepting more care responsibilities because the home health agency has limited some of its services, due to the coronavirus. Or the services are available, but I am nervous about having a parade of people into my home.

Love is laughing at oneself and seeing the humor in the situation. Love is understanding that the person with dementia is not doing things to be disagreeable; the person with dementia is trying to make sense out of a sometimes scary and nonsensical world with mixed-up memories.

Love is sometimes trying to be brave and cheerful when visiting my relative in an assisted living, plexiglass between us. Trying to explain why I can't come in and hug her. So I tell her I have a bad cold and don't want to get her sick.

Love is fighting to stay at his side while he is in the hospital, visiting restrictions be damned.

Love is becoming the memory. Love is helping to dress and bathe. Love is feeling thrilled that he put the left shoe on the left foot today. Love is feeling joy that she knows who I am today. Love is feeling triumphant because I figured out how to get him into the shower without a fight today. Love can be boastful: "Yay!! We had our first telehealth visit! Look what WE did!!"

Love is mastering ZOOM myself and helping my loved one connect with friends and family.

Love never fails, although I feel like I do at times. But where there are yucky days, and there seemed to be more this past year, they will pass. Where there are challenges, and 2020 felt like on long one, they will fade. For we know in part how to handle situations because we are learning, and every day brings more ideas and abilities than the one prior. Before I became a caregiver, I talked, thought, and reasoned differently. When I became a caregiver, I began to see the world through my loved one's eyes.

Faith, hope, and love remain. My faith gives me the strength to do some pretty difficult things. My hope helps me to persevere, because I am optimistic that this journey will continue to yield positive and surprising lessons. But it is my love for my family member, the greatest of the three, that make it all complete.

Happy Valentine's Day to the greatest examples of love: the caregivers for persons with dementia.

Summer Fun

Cinco de Maya, Memorial Day, Solstice, 4th of July, Labor Day

After being on lockdown for nearly 2 years, everyone wants to get out, visit family, and enjoy summer events. Social interaction is healthy for both caregivers (who often feel isolated) and for persons living with dementia. Here are some tips for making these events enjoyable for persons with dementia and their carers!

Safety

Yes, I know everyone wants to rip off the masks and burn them in a giant bonfire. At the time of this writing, masks are still being strongly urged for indoor events but not for outdoor events. Get vaxxed and follow the most current Centers for Disease Control and Prevention guidelines.

Helpful Hosting

If you are hosting an event and you know some of your friends or family members (who are also caregivers) are attending, here are some ways you can help them enjoy themselves.

Ask a mutual friend/family member to be the "point" person. In this case, the point person stays with or near the person living with dementia so that the caregiver can have a break. If the person living with dementia is independent but may get a little overwhelmed in social situations, the point person can "hang out" with the person and offer assistance as needed. Sometimes even individuals who are doing well may start to show anxiety or repeat themselves more frequently when in a social situation. The point person interacts calmly, offers to go with them to the buffet, or steers them to less crowded areas. Here is a great way to get someone with dementia to head to a calmer (and quieter) area: "I'm having trouble hearing with all of the people talking. Would you be OK with us going to a quieter spot?"

If the person living with dementia requires more supervision, the point person can offer to remain with the person living with dementia while the caregiver gets something to eat or drink. Sometimes, the person living with dementia "shadows" the caregiver and won't let them out of their sight. The point person can bring the goodies over to the caregiver and family member.

If you are a caregiver, you can also reach out to someone who will be attending the event and ask them for help. People are always saying, "Please let me know how I can help." People REALLY do want to help, but often do not know how. They appreciate direction!!

Timing

Everyone has their "schedule." Some people (like me) are up at 4 am and asleep by 9 pm. Others are the polar opposite. Carers should not feel bound to attend an event from beginning to end—unless it works for both them and their family member with dementia! Let's say you are invited to a 4th of July barbecue on Sunday from 1pm to 6 pm. Your family member tends to get anxious and "sundowns" around 3 pm. Let the host know your crew will be arriving at 1 pm but may need to leave at 2:30 pm, because that is the limit for your loved one. However, you can also let the host know you will "play it by ear" and stay longer if your family member is enjoying themselves!

Introductions

Everyone is always excited to see family and friends that they have not seen for some time. You can help out the person living with dementia by introducing everyone... especially family members who the person living with dementia does not see regularly. It's sad, but grandchildren who visit twice a year are more at risk for "being forgotten" than the grandchildren who pop by nearly every day. Facetime and other virtual interactions are good; but there does come a time in the severe stage where even virtual interactions may not help with recognizing family members.

Halloween

Halloween marks the beginning of the fall and winter holidays. Here are some simple ideas and tips for caregivers to have a safe and sane (ok, as sane as possible) holiday.

Play to Your Loved One's Strengths

The best way to have an enjoyable Halloween is to only do what your loved one can handle. You may already be rethinking candy distribution. Instead of answering the door holding a bowl of candy, maybe you have decided to leave candy outside of the front door. A family member with mild dementia may be able to help you to carry a plastic end table and place it a few feet from the door. Instead of leaving out a bowl of candy, you and your family member can put out a half-dozen candy bars at a time and replenish in-between the waves of Trick-or-Treaters.

On the other hand, if there is an issue with impulsiveness (especially with the frontal-temporal dementias), you may want to skip giving out candy, no matter how you decide to do it. Your loved one may be unable to stay inside while the children approach your house. They may want to hug or touch the children. It may be best to skip the trick and treating altogether.

Change Activities and Decorations

Some people living with dementia have difficulty with understanding what they are seeing. They may see a pillow and think it is a cat. Some people living with dementia have balance problems. These issues should be considered as you think about traditional activities.

Carving a pumpkin? Maybe not. Painting a pumpkin? Better idea. Also, some stores have pumpkin push decorating kits, where you stick heads and feet or other decorations into the pumpkin... think "Mr. Potato Head" but for pumpkins. Target and Walmart have cool products that produce neat pumpkin decorations but without a knife. This is also a good idea if Halloween tends to be on the warmer side, or if your area has wildlife that may munch on the pumpkins. We had a big problem with skunks feasting on our carved pumpkins when we lived in central Pennsylvania... and a bigger problem when the family dog interacted with said skunks!

Your choice around decorations may also need some tweaking. People tend to avoid decorations that may serve as an obvious trip/fall hazard. There are other decorations that may trigger a fear response. You may want to avoid the shrieking welcome mat. Or gnarly skeletal hand-in-the-candy bowl. These items can create an anxiety attack that morphs into a full-blown behavioral situation.

Some decorations can become problematic when the light changes. People living with dementia are prone to mistake innocent household items, like a coat rack or chair, for a person when the lighting changes. A creepy zombie decoration or witchy doll, no matter how cute, has the potential to be misperceived with changing light. Some families have argued with me, "But we've had that scarecrow decoration for 15 years!" True. But as the dementia gets worse, and the memories fade, the family member may not recognize the scarecrow as a beloved family Halloween heirloom.

Candy and Over-eating

Some individuals with dementia, especially frontal-temporal dementia, have difficulty with something called hyperorality: they cannot stop eating, especially sweets. This is because the "brakes" of the brain are no longer working. If you are tempted to purchase a large bag of Halloween candy from a big-box store, reconsider. Money saved is not worth the fallout when the person with dementia consumes the entire bag in one sitting. Every year at this time, I receive messages involving a person with dementia consuming 5 pounds of M&Ms in about an hour... pretty impressive, especially as the candies were in those little snack-size bags. If your loved one has that same focus on candy and sweets, perhaps give out non-food items to the Trick-or-Treaters (pencil erasers, pens, pencils—stuff you can find at the local dollar store).

Attending Fall Festivals and Parties

To attend or not to attend? That depends on the person's personality, extent of forgetfulness, and tolerance for the anticipated activity level. Some fall festivals are outside and spread out, so there is less noise and overload. Other festivals and parties can be high-volume affairs with groups of shrieking, sugar-fueled munchkins running. People living with dementia who were more on the extroverted side pre-illness may find these activities very enjoyable and even be the life of the party themselves. Others may want to leave about 5 minutes after arriving.

If you are not sure about the reaction, go to the activity but have a plan in place. Be ready to turn around and go home if the situation is overwhelming. Let the hosts know in advance that you want to give your loved one the opportunity to participate, but if he or she becomes overwhelmed, you will make a speedy exit.

Making Fall Festivals and Parties Dementia-Friendly

For those of you having or sponsoring the festivals and parties, you can help make these events a little more dementia-friendly. If possible, have a table and some chairs away from the main hub of activity. Welcome the person with dementia and the caregiver by introducing yourself. Many people who are aware of their "forgets" may avoid these situations because they don't want to embarrass themselves by not knowing names. Help out the caregiver by offering to get them some food and drink, or offer to sit with their family member while they mingle a bit. Many times, persons with dementia **shadow** the caregiver because the caregiver is their lifeline... they feel safe with that person. This creates stress for the caregiver who feels like he or she can never have a moment alone (because they can't).

Thanksgiving, Christmas, Hanukkah, Yule

Travel or Stay Home?

If the person with dementia is in the mild-to-early moderate stage and loved to travel pre-illness, traveling may be an option. As I explained in chapter 3, here are some "milestones" to help you figure out where your loved one is on the dementia continuum. If your loved one can safely and independently perform basic activities (shower/bathe by him/herself, make a cup of tea or coffee, safely use the microwave, dress in weather/situation-appropriate clothing, he or she is most likely in the mild stage. You may notice that the person does become overwhelmed and cranky in situations that were no big deal before. However, you can help with some of that behavior with good planning and back up ideas. Even airplane travel may be doable!

If the individual needs much more assistance and support to complete basic activities, for example, you have to set out the clothes or hang out in the bathroom to make sure he or she showers using soap and water, then exercise caution. If "travel" involves heading over to a relative's house in the next town, it's probably OK. If travel involves a several-hour car drive, train ride, or flight... you may want to rethink this.

Holidays: For Them or For You?

I've seen families after families push the person living with dementia beyond his or her limits because "this may be his last Thanksgiving" or "I want the grandkids to know their Mom-Mom before she gets worse." These good intentions will turn travel and the holidays into a massive nightmare. We must accommodate the person with dementia, not the other way around. The question to ask is, "How will this event affect the person living with dementia?"

For example, I dread Mother's Day when I'm working in long-term care facilities. Why? Because well-meaning families decide to take G-mom or Mom (with moderate to severe dementia) out of the Memory Care Unit and off to a crowded restaurant or family gathering. The person living with dementia is overwhelmed and frightened, becomes very anxious, and the idealized visit and plans crumble into a mess. **Here's the issue: the emotions outlive the memory!** If the annual Mother's Day outing generates fear and anxiety, the person living with dementia will remain in that state for hours after the event. The emotions then trigger other negative memories associated with those emotions, like the loss of a spouse or parent. Cue the repetitive behaviors: "I want to go home (to the childhood home)" or "Where is my mother?"

Criticisms From Others

Family caregivers cannot catch a break. Families feel guilty "leaving" their parent or grandparent in a facility for Mother's Day. It would be so much better to head to the facility and spend Mother's Day with mom in her own, safe, familiar environment. On top of their own emotions, the seagulls[2] begin their chorus. The seagulls start in on the family caregiver with statements like, "Dad should be here," "How can you be so thoughtless, you stick her in a nursing home and then you don't even have her visit on the holidays," "But she always LOVED the holidays," blah-blah-blabbity-blah. Those family members want to see Mom or Grand-Dad but do not want to go to the Memory Care Unit because of *their* own fear and guilt.

Unexpected Problems Brought Back Home

Here is another thought: if the person living with dementia is gone for several weeks, he or she may forget the map of the current home, especially if they have lived in that home for 10 years or less. I knew an acquaintance caring for her spouse with moderate-to-severe dementia. He was beginning to have problems dressing himself and bathing. She shared that that they were going to spend the holidays, traveling across the United States to visit various adult children "one last time." This couple had downsized 5 years prior and currently resided in a garden home. The wife decided they were going to spend a week in each child's home. Her spouse became more con-fused and overwhelmed with each transition. When they returned, he no longer recognized his own home. That 3-week cross-country trip accelerated his decline. His wife told me that she "wanted to make memories for the family." Memories were made for the family, but few were positive ones.

---

[2] "Seagulls" is a home health term for family members who think they know best about the care of the person living with dementia, in spite of zero involvement in day-to-day caregiving. Seagulls fly in, make a lot of noise, shit on everything, and then leave.

Holiday Travel Tips

It's a good idea to obtain a medical ID bracelet with your name and cell number. But what else to put on it? Several of my families have opted to have "diabetic" inscribed because they felt awkward with "dementia" on the ID tag. And, people with diabetes can become confused when their sugar drops. One of my caregivers simply had "brain disease" etched on the ID tag.

Traveling by car offers the most flexibility. Plan out the route with stops every 2-3 hours. Have a cooler with plenty of fluids and snacks. If your loved one needs bathroom help, you may want to stick to interstates with truck and rest stops. Another option is to look for chain grocery stores like Walmart. There are apps like "Flush," "Potty Brake," and "GoWeeWee" where you can use your smart phone to locate public restrooms. I've tried all three. Flush simply tells you if restrooms are available in your vicinity. Potty Brake and GoWeeWee allow you to search for family bathrooms. If travel involves an overnight stay, you may want to request a handicapped-accessible room. Bring something to put on the door (bells or a cheap door alarm) to wake you up if your loved one tries to exit the room.

Trains are another possibility, but get a seat in the carriage with a bathroom. Although passengers can walk from car to car, and some trains have dining and snack cars, the train is moving and this creates a fall hazard. There is also the possibility that your loved one may exit during one of the stops.

Flying... is flying. Obtain a medical pre-board, especially if you travel on airlines that do not offer assigned seats. No, you cannot sit in the emergency exit row, no matter how tempting. Many airports have family bathrooms, which is a good option if you are concerned about your loved one spending too much time in the restroom or wandering out and getting lost in the terminal. Keep connections to a minimum, if at all.

If your loved one has more issues with impulse control than with memory (behavioral-variant frontotemporal dementia, for example), or if you think the traveling experience may trigger some behaviors, have business cards at the ready that read: "My loved one has dementia and may act strangely. Thank you for your understanding and patience." You can make these business cards yourself or purchase them. Some local chapters, like Alzheimer's of Central Alabama, provide them at no charge to local caregivers.

"Rules of Engagement"

People living with dementia need to have a job and purpose.

The outlets for purpose shrink, but the need does not. Provide opportunities for the person living with dementia to help with the holiday plans. This may take some creativity on your part. For example, Mom always made the turkey. She is adamant that she is going to make the turkey. You are freaking out because last year, she sprinkled Comet on the turkey instead of salt and stuffed it with a dish towel. You have two options: tell her "no" and deal with her upset behavior, or give her a turkey to prepare. A really small one! Have another relative make and bring the actual turkey that will be consumed. Win-win.

No guessing games.

If you are going to have out-of-town guests or family members who have not seen the person living with dementia recently, give them a phone call with a quick update. They are NOT to quiz the person living with dementia; tell them to introduce themselves. If Mom knows who they are, she will laugh at them and say, "Of course you are Marty! I'd know my own son!" If Mom is having trouble keeping faces and names together, this may help prevent anxiety.

Have a buddy nearby at all times.

This is especially important with moderate to severe dementia, where the person living with dementia may need direction finding the bathroom or becomes overwhelmed with too many people. Designate a "buddy" who can hang out with the person living with dementia and move them to a quieter area if the festivities become too loud or boisterous. This also frees up the caregiver to enjoy a little break.

Avoid Peak Services.

Mass and church services are integral to many holiday celebrations. If you have options, choose the least-crowded one. This may mean attending Mass at 6 am instead of 10 AM.

If you only have one option, or you can only get to the crowded service, here are some ideas. The person living with dementia may not be able to tolerate sitting there for a couple of hours, especially if you have to arrive early to get optimal seating. I know this is against the "rules" for many congregations, but see if you can enlist someone to get there early and claim seating.

Another idea is to contact the church or synagogue NOW and ask about reserved seating for your family member. More and more faith communities have reserved seating for handicapped persons; use this seating. You may get some looks because our loved one is not in a wheelchair—so much for the scriptural passages about not passing judgment!

Have scrapbooks and photographs within reach.

This is really important if the person living with dementia begins calling relatives by the wrong name, especially if the relative is no longer living. People living with dementia move backward in time. Having scrapbooks and photographs allows everyone to see the resemblance between the person living with dementia's spouse and one of the adult children. It can also open the door to reminiscence and family history.

Bottom Line

Socialization is important, because people living with dementia and their family caregivers experience isolation. Your friends and family want to see you and support you, they just don't know how. Hopefully, you found some ideas in this chapter and will share them with your friends and family. Or suggest they all read this book!

CHAPTER 17

Sundowning: Myths and Management

Sundowning refers to behaviors seen in persons with dementia that usually occur at the end of the day. Many clinicians and caregivers/caregivers seem resigned that this will simply happen and that there is nothing that can be done to prevent or manage it... Which is why I hate the term, and prefer to think of sundowning as "tired and scared."

Where did the term "sundowning" come from?

When I worked in long-term care as a nursing assistant 30 years ago, night shift was expected to get a portion of the residents up before the end of their shift. This resulted in some people getting up at 5 or 6 o'clock in the morning and staying up for at least 12 hours. These residents would be exhausted by supper time. They would also be sitting in the common area, with other tired residents who would be crying out. The exhaustion plus the noise caused some residents to become very upset and agitated. These residents would try to leave the area (can you blame them?) Nurses and physicians who worked in long-term care noticed the uptick in these behaviors during late afternoon and early evening, and the term "sundowning" was born.

Myth #1: Sundowning always happens at sunset

Behaviors can occur at any time, and it is helpful to note patterns. Some people may show irritability and anger late in the morning, or in the middle of the afternoon. Irritability often occurs when the person living with dementia is trying to handle environmental or social demands that overwhelm the brain. In chapter 5, I use the analogy of working short-staffed. If I am trying to do my job with half of my coworkers missing, I am going to become more tired and cranky as the day goes on. I am going to make mistakes. I may even try to hit someone because I am so frustrated. A person living with dementia who is working with a large loss of brain nerves feels this way as the day goes on, or when they are placed in social situations with a lot of activity.

What to Do

Be aware of behavioral patterns. Put rest periods into the daily schedule (as long as the rest periods do not create problems with sleeping at night). Many caregivers/caregivers tell me, "She sleeps too much." When the remaining brain cells are doing two, three, or ten times the work...the person IS GOING TO BE EXHAUSTED! He may take a little cat nap after breakfast, followed by one after lunch, and may want to go to bed at 7 pm and sleep until 7 the next day. Unless there is a medical reason (like a medication that may be too sedating), go with the flow.

Myth #2: Sundowning is unavoidable. It is going to happen and there is nothing I can do about it.

I think myth #2 comes from clinicians, who just shrug when family caregivers broach this topic. I disagree. There may be some detective work that has to be done, but the detective work can help caregivers/caregivers find ways to prevent and manage the behavior.

What to Do

Again, keep track of what behavior is happening and when. Is the behavior wandering? What may be triggering it? We had a situation where one nursing home resident would sit near the door of the locked Memory Care Unit. She was usually quiet and "people watched." When my students and I began the clinical rotation, there was a delay with getting us magnetic badges so that we could unlock the doors and enter or leave. For the first week, I asked one of the staff to let us out. The students would congregate around the doors, waiting for the staff person and for me. The resident began standing with my students and becoming quite upset when she was shooed away from the door. She would yell and resist all attempts to redirect her away from the doors. The solution? The students waited over by me and we followed the staff member to the door and quickly exited, while another staff member distracted the resident with snacks.

By noting the specific behavior and pattern, you can introduce a new activity or routine prior to the event. If your family member starts pacing and wanting to go home every night at 8:30 pm, introduce ice cream at 8 pm to derail this pattern of behavior.

Clues that it May be Fear

In a later chapter about illusions and hallucinations, I describe how poor lighting, reflective surfaces, patterned surfaces, and even cluttered environments can cause people living with dementia to mis-interpret their surroundings. The wandering or agitation may be in response to something scary or disturbing to the person with dementia. However, one area that few clinicians ask about is previous violence or domestic abuse. People move backward in time as newer memories are lost but older memories become more accessible. One of my patients habitually hid in a back closet when the home became darker at dusk. Her daughter shared that this lady's first husband had been a heavy drinker and would come home after dark and begin to hurt his family. The daughter put lamp lights on timers, and the lights would come on long before sunset. The hiding behavior lessened and eventually stopped.

Myth #3: Antipsychotics are Appropriate for Sundowning

Only as an absolute last resort!!! I prefer to help family caregivers figure out what may be going on and then changing up schedules and environments. I had one spouse tell me, "Why do I have to change? He is the one with dementia!" Precisely. The person with dementia CANNOT change. You can be right, or you can be happy. I'll take happy every time.

I prefer to try antidepressants with anti-anxiety properties first. My rationale? Neurodegeneration. When brain cells die, the levels of brain chemicals goes off balance. My choice depends on the person's previous experience with antidepressants and their other health issues.

If NOTHING is working, and the behaviors are being triggered or worsened by psychotic symptoms like hallucinations, an antipsychotic may be the answer. Atypical antipsychotics like quetiapine are often the best tolerated. I avoid risperidone because of the risk for Parkinsons-type behaviors (such as problems moving or swallowing). HALOPERIDOL SHOULD BE AVOIDED!!! Haloperidol has a high likelihood of causing weird, uncontrollable behaviors like pill-rolling, lip smacking, or head rolling. It is one of the older drugs; personally, I have no idea why clinicians are using it for persons with dementia.

***

I've helped hundreds of caregivers with sundowning behavior. Contact me to find out more: rita.jablonski@gmail.com

CHAPTER 18

Dementia & Pain

"People living with dementia don't feel pain."

Bullshit. That is how I should have responded 40 years ago when I was a nursing student caring for a person with dementia in a nursing home. My patient had a foot ulcer and the physician decided to remove the top layer of the ulcer so that the wound would heal. The physician whipped out a scalpel and proceeded to cut out the top layer of the ulcer on the man's heel. I was floored. "What about giving him something for pain?" I queried, horrified at what I was seeing. The physician shook his head and blurted out, "People living with dementia don't feel pain."

People living with dementia DO feel pain: physical, psychological, emotional. They may not be able to TELL me in words about the pain. They can tell me through their actions.

Straight up, if persons living with dementia look like they are in pain, they probably are. Period. There are outdated beliefs, such as people living with dementia are less sensitive to pain, but that is utter nonsense. People living with dementia may not be able to say, "I hurt," the way you or I would. But they can communicate "I hurt" by:

- Fidgeting

- Crying

- Moaning

- Holding the body part that is hurting

- Rubbing the body part this is hurting

- Becoming rigid or restricting their own movements

- Resisting any attempt to move them by other people

- Showing agitation by pushing the caregiver away, yelling, even thrashing

Fixing the Cause

Once you realize that the person with dementia is feeling pain, the next step is to track down WHAT is causing the pain and treat accordingly.

Look first at clothing and environment. Is something rubbing? Do the shoes fit properly? Is the seat of chair intact, or is it ripped and something metal is poking the person?

Do a body scan. Do you see any angry red or swollen areas, especially the joints? Look in the mouth. Remove dentures, if the person is wearing them. Any red or white patches in there? Could be a rubbed spot or a yeast infection—both are painful.

If nothing is obvious, think about the person's health problems. Someone with long-standing arthritis may be having a flare-up. Is there a specific part of the body that the person is guarding? Could be a fracture or injury. With frailer older adults, especially women, bone fractures can happen without a fall or trauma.

This may involve a trip to the primary care provider's office to figure out the source of the pain.

Once the source of the pain is identified, the clinician is probably going to recommend pain medication. Older adults, because of changes in body fat composition and metabolism of drugs, may require smaller dosages of pain medication initially.

The available research recommends a stair-step approach. Start with non-narcotic pain-relieving medications such as acetaminophen (Tylenol) but stair-step upwards if those medications are not effective. Be careful with combination medications. For example, many "flu and sinus" preparations contain acetaminophen (Tylenol) along with other drugs. Please read the labels or ask a clinician or pharmacist for help.

Ibuprofen and naproxen can be introduced, initially at over-the-counter dosages and then at prescription dosages under the supervision of your primary care provider.

Opiates are appropriate for severe, long-term pain. Addiction is not an issue here. All of the dementias are terminal diseases. I have found that patches, such as fentanyl patches, that release constant low levels of the medication, are effective. Short-acting opiates can be used for break-through pain. The dosages of these medications can be stair-stepped upwards until the person with dementia is comfortable. I have also seen persons with dementia who have severe pain receive non-narcotics, such as antidepressants and seizure medications, in combination with the narcotics, to address certain types of nerve pain.

Non-drug therapies are also helpful and can be used in combination with drug therapies. Massage, moist heat, or cold compresses (depending on location and type of pain) can be helpful.

Sometimes clinicians shy away from the more powerful narcotic medications because of side effects like constipation or sedation. Constipation can be addressed through sufficient liquids and high dietary fiber, or psyllium supplements (e.g. Benefiber), or gentle laxatives—or a combination of all of the above, depending on the choice of narcotics. Sedation can accompany an increase in dosage but usually resolves in a day or two. If sedation remains a problem, then the dosages of the medications can be pulled back.

CHAPTER 19

Pee and Poop Problems

Constipation

Constipation is an uncomfortable annoyance for most people. When constipation occurs in people with Alzheimer's dementia or another type of dementia, it can become dangerous.

Early in my nurse practitioner career, I practiced in internal medicine. I was asked to see an elderly patient with dementia because she had "diarrhea." Her breath smelled like poop. She had vomited before coming to the office. I was shocked to feel a hard, almost rock-like, abdomen. My exam revealed a constant trickle of watery poop. This was not diarrhea. I realized that she had a life-threatening blockage in her gut and sent her to the emergency department. She had to have surgery to remove a huge blockage of poop. She died shortly afterwards. The blockage had stretched the gut so far that it tore. Poop and bacteria had spilled into the abdominal cavity and caused a massive infection.

I gently explained what happened to her family. She had a large blockage in her intestine. The gut tried to fix the blockage by constantly squeezing to get the blockage out. Picture a huge traffic accident, where only one lane of traffic slowly snakes around the pileup. The contents in her intestines started to back up, much like traffic will back up behind the accident. She had started to vomit feces, which is why her breath smelled so terrible. Her family had unknowingly made the problem worse by giving her diarrhea medication, which slowed the gut even more.

Five Ways to Fight Constipation in Persons with Dementia

People living with dementia have to be watched for constipation. They are at risk for dehydration, not eating enough fiber, taking binding medications, and holding it in.

Make Them Drink

Dementia is more than forgetting dates and facts. Dementia affects thinking and doing. Many people living with dementia may tell you they are not thirsty. Many people at the moderate to severe stage may forget how to pick up a glass and drink. If you are caring for someone with dementia, it is not enough to have the glass of water sitting in front of them. Every hour or so, pick up the glass and place it in their hands and make a "drinking" gesture. Or even better, sit with them for a couple of minutes and drink your water while giving them theirs. Popsicles, water ice, slushees, or even push-ups are other fun alternatives—especially in the summertime!

Push the Fiber

Just like people living with dementia may deny thirst, some will tell you they are not hungry. Some develop a preference for sweets and skip the veggies. One factor is that people with worsening dementia forget how to use utensils and may sit and stare at the plate. Totally unsure of what to do. This is the time to serve finger foods like grapes, carrots, and tangerine sections. Prune juice is another fan favorite. You can also dissolve psyllium (e.g. Miramax) in 6-8 ounces of liquid to sneak in some fiber. Just follow the directions for mixing.

Watch the Medications

Every time you take the person with dementia to a health care provider, ask, "Are these medications necessary?" Many medications can cause constipation, so be alert when starting a new medication. If the person with dementia needs the medication, and constipation is a possibility, work on pushing the fluids, the fiber, and daily exercise.

Schedule Toilet Time

Do not wait for the person with dementia to tell you they have to go. It may never happen, or may be too late. Even in later stages, people living with dementia may hold in the feces because they are confused and not sure where the toilet is located. I've seen situations where caregivers keep changing the undergarments but never sit the person on the commode. Practice the feel of the commode a couple of times a day, usually after eating.

MOVEMENT!

Walking around helps the gut to move, too. Physical activity is so important for many, many reasons. Now you have another one. Physical activity helps to prevent constipation.

Causes of Constipation

Not Enough Fluid in the Gut

Sometimes, people just don't drink enough water. Some people drink a lot of water, but they take water pills (diuretics). This causes water to leave the body. In warm weather, people lose fluid from sweating. No matter the cause, not enough fluid is a problem. Water is needed to keep the poops moist and slimy so that they keep moving through the gut. Without enough water, the poops become hard and slow down in the gut. Slow poops can eventually get stuck.

Not Enough Fiber

Fiber is found in fresh fruits and veggies. Picture the gut like a giant tube of toothpaste, and the gut squeezes in sections to move the poops. Fiber causes the gut to squeeze and move the poops along and out of the body. If the diet is low in fiber, the gut does not squeeze as often or strong enough to move the poops, so the poops slow down.

Medication

Some medications, like certain pain medications, can make you feel sleepy and slow. These same medications can put the gut to sleep. A sleepy gut does not squeeze the poops and move them out of the body.

Holding It In

The gut can stretch, more than the bladder. If I have to pee and I try to hold it in, eventually, I'm having an accident. The bladder can only stretch so far before it over-rides my desire to hold the pee in. The gut, however, has much more stretch to it. If I feel the urge to poop, I can hold it in and the desire will pass for a bit. If I keep holding in the poops, I can make myself become constipated.

Constipation Red Flags

It helps to pay attention, maybe keep a record, of the person's bowel movements. If the person is not pooping, and you notice vomit that smells like poop or constant trickling of liquid poop from the rectum, contact your health care provider immediately.

Preventing Poop Smearing and Poop Eating

I recently received a call from a friend who was EXTREMELY upset. She is caring for her father and he is smearing his poop all over the bathroom—towels, walls, any surface within reach. He is leaving the bathroom with feces all over his hands and clothing.

A common thread in all of the dementias is moving backwards in time. By that, I mean people forget or "unlearn" stuff in reverse of how they learned as they grew up. When their bodies are mature enough, children learn to hold their poop and use the potty, usually around age 2 ½ to 3-ish. Some children learn earlier. Some later. They learn to properly clean themselves and to wash their hands afterwards. This behavior is reinforced by parents and teachers all throughout preschool, kindergarten, and the early grades. Pooping is also known as an overlearned behavior—every time a person poops and goes through the correct steps, neural networks in the brain fire up and reinforce the connections. Properly going to the bathroom is also known as a procedural memory. Eventually, pooping becomes an autopilot activity. We do not have to exert brain power to go through the steps. One aspect about potty training that is important to think about when dealing with dementia—children are taught that pooping in their pants or having an accident is a bad and shameful thing. This is a deeply rooted memory that is reinforced throughout one's life. I will circle back to the shame issue in a bit.

As the nerve damage happens in dementia… and it does not matter which dementia… people start to forget how to do things. This forgetting is called apraxia. Apraxia is caused by breakdowns in complicated networks of neurons or brain nerve cells. At the start of the dementia, the brain tries to compensate or fix the problem by using detours to get the job done. You will see the person with dementia take longer to do things, but they are still successful. It just takes longer. As the dementia gets worse and more neurons die off, some of the necessary steps disappear. Apraxia is first noticeable with items that were most recently learned, like the most recent smartphone or TV remote. As the dementia worsens, the apraxia becomes noticeable with common appliances, like washers, dryers, ovens, and microwaves. In the late moderate to severe stages, people living with dementia have a lot of trouble performing basic care. This is where poop accidents start and poop smearing is likely to happen.

Because of neuron damage, the person living with dementia is having trouble coordinating all of the steps needed to properly poop and cleanse. They will feel the urge and start to move toward the bathroom, but then forget where the bathroom is. They may hold in the poop until they find a safe place to defecate. This can cause constipation. Some may see a bucket or trashcan and something clicks in the brain, so they use a receptacle because of the deeply rooted and subconscious fear and shame around soiling oneself. Their family members get upset because the person living with dementia pooped in the trash can that was literally next to the toilet!

The correct sequence of steps has been shuffled in the brain because of neuron loss. Some steps may be missing. This is where feces smearing can happen. The person living with dementia suddenly remembers to wipe. But they do so without toilet paper. Seeing poop on their hands, they try to cleanse but again, steps are missing. Instead of going to the sink and washing off the poop, they reflexively try to rub off the offensive poop on any handy surface. These individuals are not trying to piss off a family member or send a message. They are trying to perform a self-care activity—pooping—and are making do with the steps and memories that are readily available in their mixed-up dementia brain.

Strategies

When caring for a person living with dementia, you will need to start "spot checking" their bathroom behavior. When do you start? It depends. If the person is having trouble with urine accidents, it is time. Some families start to spot check when they find soiled underwear hidden around the house. Others start to spot check when their loved one with dementia wears the same clothes over and over again, even when the clothes are visibly soiled. Spot checking means going into the bathroom and observing the behavior or going into the bathroom and looking for signs that the person is starting to have trouble, like feces on the toilet seat.

The person living with dementia may need you to hand them the toilet paper when it is time to wipe. They may need you to give them simple and respectful one-step commands to pull up their pants and to wash their hands. Be matter of fact and kind. This is not the time to argue and fuss. The person living with dementia is not trying to upset you on purpose. In fact, they are likely very upset themselves.

As the dementia worsens, you will need to escort them to the toilet based on your knowledge of their bowel patterns. If there does not seem to be a pattern, the best option is to guide them to the toilet every 2-3 hours. Some people start to undress themselves, even in public, when they feel a full bladder or a bowel movement. It is not usually useful to ask, "do you need to use the toilet?" because you will likely receive a "no," even if they have to urinate or defecate.

Another source of fecal smearing is the use of a diaper. If the person poops in a diaper, and there is a delay in removing the diaper and cleaning off the feces, the person may experience itching or discomfort. He or she may reach into the diaper to relieve the itching, not realizing their hand is covered with feces. This is why caregivers may walk into a bedroom first thing in the morning, or after a nap, and be greeted with poop all over the place. The best way to avoid this scenario is to check the person at earlier intervals to remove the soiled diaper. Or to have them use the toilet before bedtime and before having them lay down for a nap.

Some medications have a laxative effect within a few hours of taking them. Please review all medications with your health care provider. This way, you can get the person on the toilet an hour or so after taking the medication and avoiding an accident.

What if you are trying to clean up a person living with dementia and they keep touching areas that have poop on them? Give them a towel or something to hold while you clean them up. If you have a hospital bed, tell them to hold onto the rails while you clean up. No matter how aggravated you are (and this is hard) you have to watch your tone. Yelling at them or being rough—while a very human response—is not going to make things better. It will make them upset and they may start to resist your cleaning efforts.

In some cases of dementia, the parts of the brain that tells us what is edible and what is not becomes damaged. People living with dementia may eat their own poop. I've encountered this behavior twice in my 35+ years working with older adults with dementia. The best way to avoid this situation is to put the person on the toilet when the bowel movement is likely to occur. The next best way is to remove the soiled diaper immediately. Some experts advocate the use of restrictive clothing, like adult "onesies." I understand that there are situations where the use of restrictive clothing is necessary. I'm not a fan of restrictive clothing because that means the person is sitting in feces, which can increase their risk for bladder infections and skin damage.

There are psychiatric conditions in which people "play" with poop. I am no expert in psychiatric disorders and this book is not about those disorders. This book is concerned with people living with dementia who are showing a new behavior.

Bladder Infections

Caregivers or caregivers are often surprised when their loved one with dementia suddenly becomes irritable, nasty, even physically violent. A bladder infection, also known as a urinary tract infection, may be the culprit.

Bladder Infections Often Show Up as Delirium FIRST

Any infection can create a more confused state called "delirium." People living with dementia are at high risk for delirium. Delirium can, and does, occur on top of the dementia. Think of it this way. When your body is dealing with an illness, even something as minor as a head cold, you feel yucky. Your thinking gets fuzzy. You just want to take a couple of shots of some funky-tasting medicine and go to sleep for 12 hours. Your body is so busy mobilizing its resources to fight off the infection that some of those resources get pulled away from thinking/concentrating duty. A person with dementia already has fewer neurons https://makedementiayour-bitch.com/2018/01/07/crankiness-and-irritability-in-persons-with-demen-tia/ handling thinking/concentrating/memory, so if the body pulls away even more you get WORSE confusion. And, a giant upswing in generalized irritability—which can morph into some really nasty verbal barbs and, unfortunately, escalate over time into physical assaults.

Because bladder infections (also known as urinary tract infections or UTIs) become increasingly frequent as people age, these infections go to the top of the list. Call your primary care provider and insist on being seen TODAY. You will initially run into a well-meaning front-line receptionist whose job is to "triage" the calls to determine if you REALLY need to be seen today or if you are just over-reacting. Unfortunately, some of the questions they ask (and the answers you provide) may move you to the "not urgent" list because the receptionist has not been fully trained about the workings of older adults.

Getting into the Provider's Office (or How to Deal with the People on the Phone)

When I was a nurse practitioner student, I worked in a very busy family practice site in north Philadelphia. This was before gentrification and north Philly 22 years ago was brutal. I used a padlock and chain under the hood of my car to prevent my battery from being stolen. I fielded tons of phone calls from people needing to be seen TODAY and RIGHT NOW for a variety of issues. Chest pain and drug overdoses were easy: "Call 911—Now!" But some of the other concerns required me figuring out if the situation was truly medically urgent or something else. So I get it... I'm not dissing those folks who have to make these decisions.

The front line person will ask you questions such as:

- What is your loved one's temperature?

- Is he or she having pain with urination?

- Is he or she having pain below the belly button?

- Is he or she urinating frequently?

- Does the urine smell bad?

A 30-year old with a urinary tract infection will probably report a temperature of 99 degrees Fahrenheit or higher and "yes" to all of the questions. But an 80-year-old with dementia? Or even a 63-year-old with early onset Alzheimer's dementia or FTD? Not likely. Because the front line person is not versed in how UTIs present in people living with dementia, the person may believe that your concern is not urgent and may instead schedule you for an appointment in 3 days. Or next Friday. Uh...no. If this bladder infection is not treated, your loved one can become seriously ill and die from a general body infection called sepsis.

What Number Means "Fever" in Older Adults?

The 98.6 number for "normal" body temperature was obtained by measuring the oral temperature of a couple hundred medical students (aged 21-25) and averaging it. This means that some of us have "normal" body temperatures that may be 97.6 degrees or 99.6 degrees. Our temperatures also fluctuate during the day, being lowest very early in the morning and highest in the early evening. So how would you know YOUR normal temperature? Take your temperature at the same time every day for three to four days, when you are feeling healthy—that is your baseline temperature.

The same should be done for our family members with dementia. Take their temperature every morning (before drinking a hot beverage or smoking a cigarette—both falsely raise the temperature reading) for 3-4 days. Average it. You now know their baseline temperature. I've cared for older adults with baseline temperatures as low as 96 degrees Fahrenheit. Do you see where I'm going with this?

Back to the front line person answering the phone. Your dad's baseline temp is 96. Today, it is 98.6. What the front line person does not know is a 98.6 temperature for your dad is really a 100 degree fever!

This is where you have to become really assertive and explain this to the person answering the phone!

...or respond that your dad's temp is 100 degrees and then deal directly with the provider once you see him or her. I hate to advocate fibbing but I've done exactly this when I knew that the front-line person was unable to comprehend the situation.

What About the Rest of the Questions?

Sometimes, the person with dementia will complain of pain in the lower abdominal area. Sometimes, you do notice that he or she is getting up to pee every 10 minutes. However, depending on the extent of the dementia, and if the person is incontinent of urine, the answer to the questions may be "no."

You are probably thinking, "But how do I answer the bad-smelling pee question?" Well, there is "normal" urine smell, which is ammonia-ish. Then, there is the really STRONG ammonia smell that happens with concentrated urine because of dehydration. When you urinate first thing in the morning, that is what concentrated pee smells like. Finally, there is an even stronger, yuckier smell that screams "infection." I cannot describe it but if the urine from your loved one does not fit category 1 or 2, you may be dealing with option #3.

Cool, We Got Into See the Provider! Now What?

The provider is going to ask for a urine sample. Someone will use a specially treated "dipstick" to check for evidence of a UTI. Caution, though: these dipsticks are SCREENING tools and only accurately identify infected urine about 70% of the time. The nice thing is that they are immediate and if there is evidence of an infection, the provider can prescribe antibiotics while waiting for more laboratory work. The urine should go off to the laboratory and receive a more accurate analysis. If the laboratory results indicate an infection, the next step is something called a "culture and sensitivity." The results from this procedure will tell the provider which antibiotics will be effective and which ones will not. Culture and sensitivity analyses can take at least a day or more, depending on the laboratory.

Once the UTI is treated, you should see a "clearing" of the behavior. The time it takes for the person with dementia to respond, and for the mean, nasty behaviors to go away, varies from person to person. I've seen improvement in as little as 24 hours and as long as a week.

It's Been Over a Week and the Behaviors Have Not Changed

One reason may be that the provider prescribed an antibiotic which may not be effective. Call the provider and ask about the sensitivity results. The provider may need to switch antibiotics. Another reason may be another underlying health problem. Get your loved one back in to see the provider and have a more extensive examination.

I Do NOT Want to Go Through That Again! How Do I Prevent UTIs?

1. ***Hydration, hydration, hydration.*** I am not going to give you an amount—look at the urine. Urine from a person getting enough fluids is a light yellow. Encourage non-caffeinated fluids, preferably water, all day to keep the urine a light yellow.
2. ***Spot-check bathroom habits.*** As the dementia gets worse, people forget some basic care activities. Women may forget to wipe from front to back and may do the opposite.
3. ***Support continence.*** People living with dementia start to lose motor function, meaning that they will stand up to go to the bathroom but can't make their feet work. Or they may get lost going to the bathroom. Assist your loved one to the toilet every 2 hours while awake. Don't ask, "do you have to go?" because the answer will be "no." Revisit Chapter 7 for strategies to creatively get the person living with dementia to go to the bathroom.
4. ***Change adult diapers every 2 hours.*** Adult diapers contain the same hyper-absorbent materials found in baby diapers. This is NOT

necessarily a good thing. I've seen family caregivers try to save money by changing the adult diapers once every 8 hours. I've also seen family caregivers overwhelmed by the care recipient who will NOT cooperate with removal, so the caregivers "pick their battles" and only change the soiled diapers a few times a day. Even though the urine is being absorbed and the odor may not be that noticeable, the bacteria living on the skin now have a warm, moist, dark environment to thrive and prosper in. The growing, thriving, happy bacteria are capable of moving up the urethra (where the urine travels after leaving the bladder), up into the bladder, and setting up a new home—and another bladder infection.

5. ***Cranberry juice / powder.*** There is a solid body of evidence https://www.ncbi.nlm.nih.gov/pmc/articles/PMC4863270/pdf/an011197.pdf that cranberries can protect against UTIs in child-bearing women prone to uncomplicated bladder infections. The results of studies that included older adults have been inconclusive. The ideal "dosage" of cranberry juice, or concentrated powder available in capsules, has not been determined for older adults or persons with dementia.

Helpful Hint: Talk to Your PCP About a Urine Collection Kit

One of the frustrating aspects of taking your loved one into the primary care provider's office for a urinalysis is GETTING the urine sample once you arrive. You may want to ask your PCP for the following to keep at home, so that you can obtain a urine sample and bring it with you when you and your family member go to the office. Please discuss with your PCP specific steps for properly storing the sample if an hour or more would elapse before you could get the sample into the office.

- A urine "hat" that fits in the commode to assist with urine collection.

- A plastic container for pouring the urine from the "hat."

- Cleansing wipes

- A copy of directions for correctly collecting a clean urine sample

What About Over-the-Counter Urine Dipsticks?

It depends. The majority of the over-the-counter dipsticks are designed to only check the level of white blood cells in the urine and the nitrate level. The dipsticks used by clinics and physician's offices look at more measurements, such as blood in the urine. Those "urinalysis reagent strips" can be purchased online.

Personally, I prefer to SEE patients and evaluate the situation myself in addition to obtaining urinalysis results. I do recognize that there are situations where getting the person with dementia to a provider may be nearly impossible for a variety of valid reasons. This is a conversation best had between you and your loved one's primary care provider.

How to increase water intake

It's summer, it's hot outside, and dehydration can sneak up on a person with dementia. Even "mild" dehydration can cause confusion.. and urinary tract infections (NO!!!!!!!!) How do you get a person with dementia to drink more water? Check out these ideas.

Offer Small Sips

How do you eat an elephant? One bite at a time. How do you get someone with dementia to drink more water? One sip at a time. Offering someone a huge (to them) 16 ounce or 24 ounce glass of water may trigger a "no way!" so one strategy is to hand the person living with dementia a small "dixie" cup or small juice glass with a couple of ounces of water. Do this every hour or so.

Families (and nursing home staff) often leave a large glass or container of water nearby. But people living with dementia, especially in the moderate to severe stages, do not reach out and start drinking. The nerves in the brain that coordinate the simple (to us) activity of reaching, grasping, moving the cup to the mouth, and then swallowing the liquid are not working properly. Or may be off-line completely. This is why it is important to offer frequent sips.

"But when I do that, she refuses." Approach is everything. Many of us over-talk and over-explain when we are trying to get a person living with dementia to drink. It may be more effective to simply make eye contact, smile, and place the cup or glass in the person's hand. Minimal words equal minimal refusals.

Lead by Example

In addition to handing the person water, drink your own water. Humans are social creatures. We like to eat and drink together. I personally feel awkward if I bring my lunch or breakfast to a meeting (even though we were told it was OK to do so), and no one else is eating. Social cues can remain even in the severest forms of dementia. Take advantage of those cues. Drink your water while the person living with dementia drinks his or hers.

It Does Not Have to Be Water

Water is ideal, but not everyone will drink water. Flavored waters with no sugar added are OK. You can add a couple of drops of flavoring to the water. Drinks like iced tea and lemonade can be tricky. Drinks that have caffeine cause you to pee, which defeats the whole purpose of pushing liquids. Drinks with a lot of sugar are not good... empty calories.

If the person has diabetes, sugary drinks will make them pee more. And will cause dehydration. This is because the level of sugar in the blood is already high. Once a certain level of sugar is reached, the kidney tries to "help" by pushing the sugar out of the body. The kidney dilutes the sugar with fluid. The pee looks very pale and there is a lot of it. The vicious cycle begins. The person feels thirsty, drinks more soda, and the kidney "helps" by pushing the sugar out of the body in the form of pee. Bad situation.

Is Soda Ever OK?

Sometimes. This is where you weigh the pros and cons. If my 85-year-old aunt will ONLY drink ginger ale and she does not have diabetes, I'm not going to fight that fight. If she prefers orange soda, I may cheat by cutting her beloved Fanta with some seltzer water or **lots of ice cubes, which will melt and dilute the soda.**

Speaking of ice cubes, see how your loved one feels about cold liquids. Some people have no problem with cold items but as we age, the gums in our mouth shrink a bit. This opens the sensitive tooth root to cold liquids and foods. Some people cannot tolerate cold (or hot) liquids because of sensitive teeth. If that is the case, serve liquids that are cooler but not cold.

Popsicles and Freezer Pops

Yes, frozen water is just as good as liquid water. Pay attention to sugar content if the person has diabetes (or is at risk for diabetes). Use popsicles with no added sugar. Or, make your own. I found popsicle molds in several stores. Pour the lightly flavored liquid, such as homemade decaffeinated iced tea, into the molds. Freeze. Serve!

Foods with Lots of Liquid

Another way to sneak in fluid is by eating. Watermelon is the first fruit that comes to mind —and it's delicious! Cantaloupes, tomatoes, and grapes are other options. Jello works, too!

***

I am really good at helping family caregivers easily and creatively handle (and prevent) many of these behaviors. Reach out and find out how I can help you: rita.jablonski@gmail.com

CHAPTER 20

Driving

When Is It Time to Stop?

Depends on the answers to the following questions:

1. Any recent accidents or "near-misses"?
2. Any new damage showing up on the car?
3. Is the person with dementia getting lost in familiar places?
4. Any impulsive or road-rage behaviors?
5. Would you feel comfortable riding as a passenger if the person with dementia were driving?
6. Would you feel comfortable having your child or grandchild as a passenger if the person with dementia were driving?

A "yes" response to #1, #2, #3 or #4 suggests that the person should not be driving. I put in #4 because I've had experiences with persons with frontal lobe problems who became overly aggressive; I recognize that a "yes" to #4 would apply to many people without a dementia diagnosis. A "no" response to #5 or #6 is a definite NO THE PERSON SHOULD NOT BE DRIVING. I guess you could make the argument that any driver, regardless of cognitive abilities, getting a "no" to #5 or #6 has no business behind the wheel of a car.

What if there are no problems right now and no concerns?

This is a little trickier. In the clinic, I recommend limiting the trips to local, well-known places that the person has driven to for years (supermarket, barber shop, hair salon, church); no highways; only during daylight; and only during good weather. It is a good idea for someone to be a passenger on a regular basis to make sure the driving is still OK.

I completely understand how important personal freedom is to all of us, especially persons with dementia. But if a person with dementia is unaware of his or her driving problems, you are going to have to take away the keys. In some cases, remove the car because hiding or removing the keys is often not enough.

Bottom Line

If you have questions or concerns about whether or not a person with dementia should be driving, talk to your primary care provider, a clinician (physician, nurse practitioner, physician's assistant) experienced with dementia care, or even local law enforcement.

Taking Away the Keys

I offer some suggestions that I have used, or other family caregivers have used, to end driving. *The worst thing you can do (in most cases) is to hold a "family meeting" and explain to mom or dad why everyone wants them to stop driving. If the person with dementia is unaware of their memory problems and driving issues, this approach will get you nowhere!*

1.   **Take a "break" from driving.** In my practice, I often tell the person with dementia (Person living with dementia) that I want him or her to "take a break" from driving until I can see them again (3-6 months later). Most times, the Person living with dementia is unaware that he or she has memory problems and will hotly deny it if someone brings up the topic. I try to use a physical, non-threatening reason for the "break" (see #2). **Think about it: what feels better to you, "Give up chocolate for a couple of months" or "You can never have chocolate again"?**

2. **Use a physical reason for the driving "break."** As we age, we have more and more physical problems that could create driving issues. If the person has any physical limitation that could REMOTELY pose a problem, I use that. Some examples include neck pain (*Since you can't turn your neck, take a break from driving until we get that fixed*), hip or knee problems, and even foot

numbness from diabetes. Six weeks after my right knee replacement, my son accompanied me while I drove around. I thought my driving was fine, but he had concerns about my reaction time and use of the pedals. I stopped driving for 3 more weeks until my reaction time improved. Now, if you had told me I needed to stop driving because of my memory...

If #1 and #2 don't work:

3. Disable the vehicle. Depending on the year, make, and model of the car, this can be done in a variety of ways. For cars that use the electronic fobs (keyless), remove the battery (or have the dealer do this). For older makes and models, disconnect the battery cables. I'm sure there are other ways to disable vehicles; my family caregivers never cease to amaze me with creative ways to render the vehicle non-driveable. **One caveat:** I had one situation where the patient with dementia asked a neighbor to look at her car, and the helpful neighbor reconnected the battery cables. So, if you go this route, you may want to let the "helpful neighbors" know what is going on.

4. Remove the vehicle. One family member told his dad that the car needed some recall work. He drove the car over to another family member's house and placed it in the garage. For a couple of weeks, dad asked about the car and the response was, "It is still in the garage getting work done." Ultimately, dad stopped asking about the car. Many other creative family members used variations on the theme of "the car is getting work done." No matter how tempting, DO NOT tell the Person living with dementia that the car has been stolen. You will cause feelings of fear and anxiety, which is not only a crappy thing to do but these feelings may trigger a domino-effect of other emotions. Or the Person living with dementia may report the car stolen and YOU have created a ginormous mess!

***

Check out my videos on this topic: https://makedementiayour-bitch.com/videos/

CHAPTER 21

Firearms

After one of my law enforcement talks, a group of investigators approached me with some troubling stories. Not only were they struggling with on-the-job dementia issues, all were dealing with this disease personally. I've changed some details to maintain confidentiality... however, if these stories sound familiar, it is because the problem is WAY more prevalent even though it is well hidden.

"My Uncle Reported the Guns as Stolen."

One law enforcement officer was visibly frustrated. His uncle was diagnosed with "some type of dementia" in a rural town in Alabama. Guns are serious business here in Alabama, by the way. The man's family removed all weapons and ammunition from the house. My cousins told him constantly, "Dad, we have to take these guns out of the house." Dad had minimal short-term memory. In his world, his valuable guns were missing. In his Dementia Land, the obvious reason for the missing artillery was theft. Dad called the police and reported the guns as stolen.

"...and then, the deputies arrived."

He continued to share that his uncle was "having a good day" and his complaint seemed authentic to the officers on the scene. The family spoke to the officers privately and explained the situation: their father's judgment was "off" and he was shooting the guns on the property without taking any safety precautions like limiting his shooting to a designated area that had been fortified with backstops. The officers were not sure how to proceed. Was this the case of a family trying to protect others, or was this a case of elder exploitation? The officers took custody of the firearms and handed the situation over to a detective for further investigation. After a lengthy process, where one of the family members was initially charged with theft, the situation was resolved and all charges were dropped.

The officer telling me about the situation just stood there, shaking his head. Other participants were listening in and nodding. Some had been on calls just like this one. I did not have any easy, pat answers. I did have suggestions that I shared with them, and that I am sharing with my readers.

Suggestions for Family Members

When a family member is diagnosed with dementia, there is often feelings of being overwhelmed. So much to take in; so much to do. However, handling these issues early is an act of kindness to your future self!

Preemptively contact local law enforcement about the situation. Ideally, have at least 2 family members go together. This looks less like a single family member trying to take advantage of an older adult. Sad, but elder exploitation is a reality.

Bring documentation from a health care provider. The provider may not be comfortable disclosing the exact diagnosis—this is a HIPAA issue—but the provider may be able to convey the severity of the problem by using general terms. One approach is to write, "The individual has a neurodegenerative condition that is causing problems with judgmen and I advised the family that she should not have access to firearms for safety reasons." By the way, this wording can also be used to document that the individual should not be driving, should not have access to power tools, or should not be handling finances.

If this has not been done already, contact an experienced attorney (ideally, someone well-versed in elder law) to obtain a power of attorney. This way, you have some documentation if the person with dementia accuses you of stealing money or inappropriately handling finances.

Suggestions for Law Enforcement

No, it is not your job to determine the diagnosis. You are trying to make sense of the situation. Speak to the person making the complaint and listen carefully. Observe the mannerisms and speech patterns. One thing I stress when I work with law enforcement is that the individual may not appear like a stereotypical "old person with memory problems." If you are dealing with a person who has a type of frontal-temporal dementia or early onset Alzheimer's disease, that person will be on the young side.

As you interact with the person making the complaint, listen for repetition. Not the obvious, "who are you?" but more subtle repeats. For example, the individual may repeat a sentence like "I just don't understand why my family is acting this way," three, four, or maybe five times in a 10-minute interaction. To experienced officers and investigators, the repetition is going to exceed the usual repetition individuals may offer when stressed-out. I know this is a qualitative judgement call.

Also, listen for content that is all over the place. The complaint turns into a complicated story, and you have to keep bringing the focus back to the issue at hand. You may also observe inappropriate laughing or attempts at humor.

Another idea is to request that the person making the complaint write out what happened. Your script can be, "I want to make sure I get everything right." The caveat here is that this strategy is only useful if the person is literate. While not foolproof or diagnostic, this activity may provide valuable information. Does the printing or handwriting get smaller and smaller? Does the written description follow a logical pattern? Or is it all over the place and not really making sense? Is the person unable to do it at all? Does the individual ask repeatedly, "Now, what is it that you wanted me to do?" This task may help you to see possible issues around attention, concentration, and following direction that you would not have seen if you had just interacted verbally.

"We left the guns, but removed all of the bullets."

I've had some family members go this route. In fact, the first time I heard it I thought it was a very creative approach. By removing the ammunition, and leaving the firearms, the person living with dementia was less likely to fuss at the family members. Conflict avoided!

But what happens when the person with dementia answers the door *holding a firearm?* Or is walking around outside with the hunting rifle? Nobody else knows that the gun may be empty. Law enforcement arriving on scene are encountering a person with a weapon. This is not going to end well.

Stay tuned...

I started working with first responders in 2018. I have provided dementia crash courses: types of dementia, common behaviors they may encounter, and basic strategies for dealing with repetition, refusal, delusions, and some other behaviors. First responders are HUNGRY for this information. My work with law enforcement is now a personal mission. In late 2020, my son graduated from Florida Highway Patrol's Academy, and he is currently a trooper in Manatee County. He periodically calls me after a shift and relays an interaction with a person likely living with dementia. I continue to use my knowledge and experience to help him figure out ways to safely and effectively work with people living with dementia. I intend to develop more programs that help first responders become more dementia-friendly.

***

If you are a first responder, contact me for live group training. I'm funny as f*ck and I know my shit. Plus, as a nurse with 2 kids in law enforcement and a bunch of family members who are firefighters, I am part of the first responder family—so you will get the family discount!

--rita.jablonski@gmail.com

CHAPTER 22

Wandering

People living with dementia wander for a variety of reasons. Many times, the wandering behavior is a reaction to an unrelated event—that is, people living with dementia do not simply decide to go on a journey. Some people are at higher risk for wandering than others. Read on for the reasons behind the wandering behavior, some of the signs of beginning wandering behavior, and how to prevent/manage it.

Why Do People Living with Dementia Wander?

Lost in Their Own Home

When we live somewhere, our minds create a map of the location. If we relocate, and most of us do, our minds create new maps of our new location. The new maps literally overlay the older maps. Sometimes, the maps can become mixed up. Have you ever reached for a light switch and realized you were reaching in the wrong place? This usually happens when you have recently moved to a new place but your mind is still accessing the former map. The more one moves, and the shorter the time between the moves, the more likely the location maps get intertwined. I have experienced this first hand. Because of job changes and a couple of other life events, I have lived in 5 different houses since 2012. I've been in my most recent place 7 months, and I still open the wrong cabinet to locate my coffee mug.

People living with dementia may literally get lost going to the bathroom because of mixed-up mind maps. As the dementia worsens and the brain shrinks, the person with dementia moves backward in time. He or she may lose the layout of the CURRENT house or apartment. Instead of turning left to head towards the bathroom, he or she may turn right and find themselves outside. Usually, the person will turn back and head into the house, but if the door should close behind them and lock the person may panic and try to seek help and wind up completely lost because he or she no longer possesses the neighborhood map. Or, the mind may be accessing the wrong neighborhood map and the person becomes hopelessly lost within a few feet of their current home.

Ever lose or misplace something valuable? I have... and I have spent hours searching for it. I have been so engrossed in the search that I suddenly found myself looking in the strangest places. The person with dementia may be looking for something, or someone, and find themselves outside. Although it defies OUR logic, to them it may make sense to keep searching OUTSIDE of the house. The person may be so engrossed in the search that he or she does not realize they are becoming lost until it happens.

Leaving a Stressful Situation

I had a relative who handled all stressful situations by "going for a walk." It did not matter the time of day or the weather. When she became overwhelmed, off she went. There were times when she and her spouse were engaged in a heated argument and she simply walked out for an hour or two. She always came back. This was her method of coping and she used it her entire life.

When she developed beginning signs of dementia, she still used this coping method... but she sometimes returned to the house with help from a neighbor or a police officer. We started to recognize that if *something made her anxious, she would fidget, then pace, then attempt to leave the room.* As the dementia progressed, she continued to use a decades-old coping pattern but she no longer had sufficient memory to safely find her way back.

Repeating a Life-Long Pattern

We are creatures of habit. We tend to repeat the same activities on a daily basis. Some of us may even have a favorite or habitual breakfast or snack. These habits and patterns provide comforting structures to our lives.

When someone has dementia and moves backward in time, he or she may fall into an old groove. He or she may believe they have to leave to go to work, or to pick up the children. As the brain shrinks and the newer memories are lost, the older deeper memories literally rise to the surface and may seem very real. Sometimes the activities of others may accidentally "cue" or "trigger" these memories and their related behaviors. For example, one of the nursing home residents for whom I cared was a retired nurse. Shift-change was a trigger for her to try to leave the building because she saw the nurses putting on their coats and exiting the unit. She happily tried to exit with the group and she became upset when she was told she could not leave.

Who Is At Risk for Wandering?

Honestly, anyone with a memory problem and who can move independently, even in a wheelchair, is a wandering risk. But some people are more at-risk for this behavior than others:

People Who Were Always Active

There are individuals who literally rarely sat still their entire lives. My mother, for example, is always on the move. She raised five children as a single parent and worked multiple jobs. I only ever saw her sit still in one of 3 places: church (and even then, she was sitting, standing, kneeling throughout the Mass); at the dinner table for meals (15 minutes maximum, and then she was jumping up and down to get an item, turn off the stove, or put something back in the fridge); or on the commode (don't judge—for the longest time we only had one bathroom in the entire house.) Even now, in her mid-seventies, she buzzes around her house like a bee on crystal meth. If she should ever develop dementia, she will be a HUGE wandering risk.

People Who Walked or Ran as Exercise or as a Coping Mechanism

Like my relative, people who used walking or running as their preferred activity or in response to stress are likely to continue those movement behaviors even as their memory begins to unravel.

Recent Relocation

Relocation for a person with dementia can create a wandering issue. Sometimes, relocation cannot be helped; the person with dementia requires a safer space, or the adult child caregiver has to move mom or dad back to the caregiver's home in order to fulfill care-giving responsibilities. However, I have seen situations where a person with moderate to severe dementia is taken on a trip and becomes horribly disoriented in the hotel or in the host's house and leaves the area looking for "home."

Care-Recipient/Caregiver Learning Curve

Not all of us are wired to be caregivers or caregivers. Just like all of us can sing but only a minority of us are singers, all of us can be caring but a much smaller subset can be true caregivers. **THIS IS NOT A JUDGMENT, IT IS REALITY.** Yet, many of us become caregivers or caregivers "by default" because we are a spouse, a sibling, a friend, or an adult child of someone with dementia. Some people are able to intuitively "figure things out" and provide care in such a way that the person with dementia does not feel anxious. The MAJORITY of us have to learn (and you are reading this book, which means you are trying to learn!!). Caregivers who are new to the situation, or who are struggling, may not realize that the person with dementia is much more impaired than he or she looks (or tries to act), and may not provide sufficient supervision. Caregivers also worry about being too overprotective and not respecting the person with dementia's autonomy and dignity. That is a valid concern, and I address it in other blog posts. Caregivers may be unwittingly triggering anxiety in the person with dementia by arguing, talking too much, or constantly presenting OUR reality. Faced with anxiety, the person with dementia attempts to leave the stressful situation by going out the door.

Strategies to Prevent Wandering

Provide Daily Physical Activity

People who crave activity are not going to change. Accompany them on their walks or enlist the help of a responsible person to do so. Do not rely solely on animals. I cared for a gentleman whose family had him take the family dog for a walk every day. Their rationale was that the dog would always find its way home. True. The dog did always find its way home, but not always with the gentleman on the other end of the leash.

Some caregivers take their loved one to the gym and have them use the treadmill. In fact, one of my friend took her 88-year-old mother to the gym daily, and she used a treadmill without incident or injury. He even had her weight-training. My friend credits this activity with her mother's improved outlook and physical functioning. I have caregivers who participate in water aerobics with their loved ones with dementia. It does not matter how you move... just move!

Strategically "Hide" Exits

Amazon sells murals that look like bookshelves but stick onto doors. These murals work. I first saw one in a local long-term care facility and thought, "Wow, what a cool idea!"

Child-Proof Door Handles

One of my family caregivers purchased plastic doorknob covers that had to be squeezed a certain way in order to open the door. They were designed to keep children from exiting rooms. These child-proof handles also worked with the family member with dementia. A word of caution, though... if the person with dementia is trying to leave the and the doorknob will not work, agitation and anger may arise. I would prefer that people go with camouflaging exits.

Other Safety Tips

Check with your local Alzheimer's Association or Area Agency on Aging to see if law enforcement participates in any type of wandering program.

Some areas provide free or low-cost GPS-style bracelets that can be used to track someone with dementia if they become lost. Another option is to make sure that the person has a Medic-alert bracelet with "Dementia" printed on it and the caregiver's cell phone. Some family members enable the "Find my Phone" app on smart phones. That only works if the person keeps the cell phone on his or her person at all times. They usually do not.

***

I provide monthly free webinars. <u>Subscribe to my newsletter to learn more!</u>

Or use the QR code:

CHAPTER 23

Handling "Rage" Behavior in Persons Living with Dementia

We all get angry. At ourselves, at others, at situations. Most of us have enough brain power and insight to read other peoples' faces and body language and realize we just messed up. Or we were out of line. Or maybe we were justified in having the anger, but not in acting out. This awareness and insight can be lost as the frontal lobe, prefrontal cortex, and other parts of the brain shrivel away when dementia worsens.

Imagine that you wake up and you do not recognize the room. You get out of bed, wondering where you are. Your spouse appears. Relieved, you ask your spouse, "Why aren't we at home?" Your spouse tells you that you ARE at home. "How can that be?" you ask. Your spouse seems impatient with you. You sit down in a chair and there is the TV remote. You try to turn on the television—nothing works. You try taking out the batteries, but now… the batteries do not fit into the remote anymore. Your spouse puts down a cup of coffee and you show them the remote.

"Dammit, that is the sixth time today you took those batteries out."

What? You just woke up! How dare you be talked to that way!! You are getting angry. "No its not!!" you yell.

Your spouse hands you back the remote. You push the buttons, but again, nothing works. You look up, and your spouse sighs, then takes the remote. IT WORKS!! You wonder, how come the remote works for them but not for you???

You try to follow the television program but it makes no sense. You try to change the program but the sound goes away. You try to increase the sound, but now the screen is blank. No, wait. There are words: "Input 3 unavailable." What does that mean?

You get up to find your spouse. You search for hours. You are getting very, very upset. Why are you alone? Finally, you see your spouse in one of the rooms putting away laundry.

"Where have you been?" you ask. "I haven't seen you for hours!"

Your spouse looks at you in a confused and sad way. "I've handed you the TV remote 15 minutes ago. I've been here in this bedroom since then."

The above scenario describes how people living with dementia, especially those who are not aware that they have memory problems, find themselves in a nightmarish world where the meaning of time changes; where they wake up in a house that is obviously not their home, yet everyone is telling them the opposite; and where simple, everyday objects no longer work for them—but seem to work for everyone else. Step into their shoes for a minute:

The world does not make sense. Everyone is telling me I'm wrong... but I'm not!! I'm trying to meet my needs and live my life, but I'm constantly in trouble. And everyone is talking "at" me. All I hear is "no." I'm not stupid and I'm not a child, but I'm starting to feel like I'm guilty of being both.

It's no surprise why many people living with dementia easily become angry, and why some people living with dementia fly into a rage. Anger and rage seem to be more of an issue in persons living with bvFTD, but it can show up in any of the dementias. If you have a loved one who frequently shows anger, you may want to try some of these strategies.

The "OK and" / "OK I hear you" Approach

In the example above, the person living with dementia keeps getting information that is not aligned with their immediate experience. You can imagine how this constant flow of wrong (in their world) information can create anger. Two ways to acknowledge what they are saying without triggering anger is the "OK and" or "OK, I hear you" approach. I've always been an advocate of using "OK" as a way to let the person living with dementia know that I've heard them. However, I would always follow with a "but." A couple of years ago, I read an excellent book by Susan Scott titled "Fierce Conversations." She suggested using the word "and" instead of "but" in difficult conversations to present two co-existing realities. For example, my boss wants me to take on another time-sensitive project while I'm getting ready to go on vacation in two days. If I respond, "you want me to take on this project but I'm leaving for Italy in two days," it sounds like I am telling my boss there is my reality and then there is her reality. On the other hand, if I say, "You want me to take on this project and I'm leaving for Italy in two days," the message and vibe change. I am presenting two, equally valid situations. I've used this technique to successfully handle many work-related conversations. It works to reduce anger, too. Let's look at a typical anger-producing conversation.

Person living with dementia (PLwD): "I really think I should be driving again."

Caregiver (CG): "No, you should not. The doctor said you should not be driving."

PLwD: "I'm fine! I am the safest driver around. I've never had an accident in 50 years of driving."

CG: "No, you are not. You had 3 speeding tickets last year. You cannot safely drive. You drive too fast and you don't pay attention."

PLwD (obviously angry at this point): "What do you know? I'm fine, I can drive. I'll show you. Give me the keys and I'll show you that I can drive!"

At this point in the conversation, the caregiver is screwed. If the caregiver appropriately refuses, the anger escalates to the point of rage. If the caregiver hands over the keys, game over.

This is how to apply both the "OK and" and the "OK, I hear you" strategy:

PLwD: "I really think I should be driving again."

CG: "OK, and the doctor said you should not be driving." *Notice how the "OK and" shortened the sentence and shifted the blame to the doctor. It's always better for the caregiver to be the "good" person and let others be the heavies!*

PLwD: "I'm fine! I am the safest driver around. I've never had an accident in 50 years of driving."

CG: "OK, and I understand you are upset." *It is tempting to present reality to the person living with dementia. In situations where the person living with dementia is known to quickly become angry to the point of rage, it is best to avoid arguing.*

PLwD: "Yes, I'm upset. I'm upset because I should be driving."

CG: "OK, I hear you."

The second conversation demonstrates how the caregiver acknowledges that they have heard the person living with dementia. The caregiver skillfully uses the "OK and" strategy to explain the situation without triggering anger by using the dreaded "no" word. The caregiver also uses "OK, I hear you" to validate that they are listening and paying attention to the person living with dementia.

The caregiver in the second conversation did not argue. As noted in previous chapters, arguing and logic do not work in Dementia Land. This is because OUR logic is not THEIR logic. Their perspectives are altered by the brain damage caused by their specific dementia.

You Can Be Right or You Can Be Happy

Caregivers often say to me, "Why do I have to change? Why do I have to watch my words?" Simple. YOU can change and adapt—THEY cannot. You can be right. You can argue and tell the person with dementia how wrong, how dangerous, and how f–ed up they are. Don't be surprised by the surge or rage that is unleashed.

Instead, you can adapt your communication style to compensate for their brain damage. When I advise you to adapt your communication style, I mean your total communication style. We communicate verbally and nonverbally. For people living with dementia who are prone to anger and rage, it is very important to monitor your facial expressions. Try to keep your expressions positive or neutral. Just like you have to avoid overt verbal disagreement, you need to avoid showing disapproval or disagreement through your non-verbal cues.

Safety is important

In cases where the person living with dementia is prone to anger and rage, make safety preparations. First, alert local law enforcement that your loved one has dementia. There may be specific safety programs designed for persons living with dementia and their caregivers. Be prepared for a "worst case" scenario, like you are locked out of your house by the person living with dementia or you may have to leave immediately without getting your cell phone, money, wallet, or purse. You may want to have an overnight bag with an extra charger, a cheap cell phone (that you have already programmed with your contacts), a change or two of clothes, alternative ID (such as your passport or military ID), credit card, extra set of house keys, and some cash, either locked in your vehicle's trunk or stashed with a close friend and neighbor. Your vehicle should be parked so that you can make an immediate departure, such as in the driveway instead of the garage, or backed into the parking lot so that you can pull out easily.

Unfortunately, I have encountered situations where the anger and rage from a person living with dementia caused the caregiver harm. If the person living with dementia is extremely angry and is trying to leave, do not try to physically stop them if you may get hurt. This is especially important if the person living with dementia is physically larger and stronger than the caregiver. Let them leave. They may simply walk around the property or pace in front of the house. After some physical movement, they may return to the house calmer. If they do leave the property, you can notify law enforcement to assist with locating them.

CHAPTER 24

Caregiver Topics: Back-Up Plan

Caregivers for persons living with dementia need a back-up plan. There needs to be someone who can temporarily or permanently care for the person living with dementia. Best to plan for the situation now, rather than scramble under difficult situations.

Medical Emergencies

Caregivers are familiar with medical emergencies involving their loved one. But what if the caregiver suddenly has a heart attack? This situation is becoming more common, especially among spousal caregivers. The spousal caregiver often ignores his or her own health needs because of the all-consuming nature of caregiver. "I can't deal with one more thing right now." But then the caregiver's body reaches a limit, and the health care issue takes center stage.

One creative caregiver placed signs throughout his house:

To Emergency Workers (Fire, Police, Paramedics):

My wife has dementia and can not be left here alone. She either comes with me to the hospital or stays with one of these people:

Kathy (daughter): 205-555-3371

Melanie Roberts (neighbor): 205-555-1690

He placed these signs on the refrigerator, over his bed, and on the front door inside of the porch. He even provided this information to his local police precinct and fire house.

Urgent Healthcare Needs

It breaks my heart seeing caregivers dragging oxygen tanks into the clinic. I know of caregivers who have multiple physical problems but continue to provide intense, hands-on care to their loved ones living with dementia. These caregivers delay important tests and procedures. If you recognize yourself in this blog, please start putting together a respite team. If you have access to in-home care through your state's Medicaid program, sign up and start using it. Reach out to your families, be they biological, by choice, or by faith. Please do not assume that others will say "no." If you know of people in this predicament, offer help. It can be as basic as going with the caregiver to the appointment and keeping the person living with dementia occupied.

Legal Paperwork

A power of attorney pertains to financial matters, period. Too many people believe that a "power of attorney" makes them legal guardians for people living with dementia. No, it does not. Most hospitals and long-term care facilities do not demand proof when a caregiver announces that he or she is the decision-maker. However, if two or more individuals assert that they are the decision-makers and the decisions are different, problems happen. It is best early in the dementia journey to have a living will and healthcare proxy. The living will describes what life-saving measures the person living with dementia is willing to accept and under what circumstances. The healthcare proxy identifies the MEDICAL decision-maker. Honestly, everyone should have a living will and healthcare proxy.

I asked about a living will and healthcare proxy while working with a woman with mild dementia. She shrugged and simply said, "My children will make the best decision when the time comes. I trust them." Her two adult daughters looked at her with pained expressions. This was not helpful. I gently explained that she was going to cause her daughters guilt unless we talked about some options today. We did. I think more clinicians need to be a bit assertive in these types of situations.

Click here for more information on advance care planning. https://makedementiayourbitch.com/2017/10/06/the-3-questions-every-dementia-caregiver-should-ask-clinicians-starting-the-palliative-care-conversation/

Death

Caregivers seem to assume that they will outlive https://makedementiayourbitch.com/2018/12/11/parents-caring-for-adult-children-with-dementia/ the person living with dementia. Some caregivers go to great lengths to minimize the seriousness of the situations. These caregivers do not want to burden adult children. Or, they want to preserve the dignity of the person living with dementia by hiding deficits or care needs. These desires are understandable. But one day, the caregiver dies and the remaining family members are unprepared for the amount of care the survivor requires. In fact, the adult children may believe Dad is "just a little forgetful" and they unwittingly place him in an unsafe situation by leaving him alone with no supervision or support. Meanwhile, Dad has no ability to prepare meals or even dress appropriately. Utilities are shut off and a neighbor discovers Dad collapsed outside, dehydrated and covered in filth.

Caregivers should be having honest conversations now about the needs of the person living with dementia. Just like parents select individuals to raise their children if the unthinkable happens, so must caregivers select alternative caregivers. If there is no one to take over, then the caregiver should make arrangements with a memory care facility or nursing home. This sounds cold, but if adult protective services becomes involved, placement will happen... at the first available facility, not the preferred facility.

Bottom Line

All of us prepare, to some extent, for the unexpected and unwelcome. Dementia caregiving is no exception.

CHAPTER 25

Can a Person Living with Dementia Safely Make Decisions?

Several years ago, my clinical practice included covering an assisted living facility. I was called to evaluate a new resident who was complaining of chest pain. Mrs. Q had had heart attacks in the past; I wanted to send her to the local hospital for an evaluation. Mrs. Q also told me that she wanted to go to the hospital. When I spoke with her granddaughter, who was also her health care proxy, I was told:

"I think she has indigestion. She also has dementia, so she doesn't know whether or not she wants to go to the hospital."

After a lengthy conversation, the granddaughter reluctantly agreed to meet Mrs. Q at the hospital. Turns out, Mrs. Q *was* having a heart attack and it was severe. She was admitted to the hospital.

A few days later, I called the granddaughter to check on Mrs. Q. The granddaughter was extremely angry and frustrated. Mrs. Q was not eating, and a surgeon was pushing for a feeding tube. The granddaughter had walked into the room as the surgeon was speaking with Mrs. Q, who was upset and was telling the surgeon, "NO!"

"I asked my grandmother, 'Do you want a feeding tube put in your stomach?' She said, 'No.' So I told the surgeon to leave. Yes, I know she has dementia, but she still knows what she wants and what she doesn't want."

I was floored. **When Mrs. Q's opinions differed from that of her granddaughter, the grand-daughter quickly used the dementia diagnosis to ignore Mrs. Q's choices. When Mrs. Q's choices and opinions mirrored those of the granddaughter, the granddaughter believed that Mrs. Q had the capacity to make decisions.**

I started paying more attention to how family members judged the decisional abilities of people living with dementia. Sure enough, I began to see the same pattern. Family members who agreed with their loved one's decision, or who benefited from the outcome, were likely to agree that the person living with dementia had intact decisional capacity—they were able to make a sound decision even with the dementia going on. Family members who did not agree with their loved one's decision, or who felt that they were not going to benefit from the outcome, were likely to dismiss their loved one's opinion on the grounds of dementia.

Here is the bottom line: the ability to make a decision is not an "on/off" light switch. It is more like a gradual dimmer and must be evaluated for each individual and for each circumstance. How do you know if someone living with dementia has the decisional capacity for a specific problem or situation? These 5 questions can start the conversation rolling. Caregivers will probably have other related questions for each of the big ones.

1. Tell me about the decision. (*What is the decision? What does it mean to you?*)

2. If you go through with _____, what may happen?

3. Tell me who your decision may help.

4. Tell me who your decision may hurt.

5. Is someone or something "pushing" you to make this decision?

One must evaluate the responses based on how severe the dementia is. I probably would not ask these questions of someone with moderate to severe dementia. The asking of the questions is a process; we are providing an opportunity to really find out what the other person is thinking. On one hand, we want to protect our loved ones from financial abuse or unsafe conditions.

On the other hand, we want to respect their autonomy.... their ability to make their own decisions.

Let's say I have a parent with dementia who is living in his own house. One of the adult children wants that parent to move in with her. The parent steadfastly refuses. Here are his responses to the questions:

"My daughter wants me to move in with her, but I don't like where she lives. It is not close to where my friends are and I'll never see them. If I move in with her, I'll have to sell my house and I will always be a 'guest.' I will never have my own place. Moving in would help my daughter, she would not have to drive over here to check on me. True, I'll be with someone but she works every day so I'll still be by myself while she is at work. It would be nice to have company every evening. I feel like my children are pushing me to move so that they won't have to worry about me."

Now, the reality is that the move is not a question of "if" but a question of "when." At least the parent is sharing some of his concerns about feeling homeless and becoming a permanent house guest. His daughter may be able to come up with some compromises based on this conversation. Perhaps it would be better if he were to relocate to an apartment in a senior community or to an assisted living environment; this may not have occurred to the adult children as a possibility because they were so focused on one potential "solution" to their concerns about their father's safety.

These five questions can also be useful in checking to see if the person living with dementia is refusing care, medication, or some other necessary item due to true autonomy or instead, due to refusals based on dementia or fear.

Decisional Capacity versus Decisional Competence

What is the difference between decisional capacity and decisional competence?

Financial exploitation is a real problem that impacts persons living with dementia and their families. Families struggle with balancing independence with providing safety.

Decisional capacity is the ability to make a decision and can be evaluated by a clinician, such as a nurse practitioner, physician, social worker, or psychologist. Decisional capacity is situational. That is, a person may have the ability to make a decision about wanting someone listed as a healthcare proxy. However, that person may lack the decisional capacity to decide how to safely invest retirement funds. This book is all about dementia, so I'm discussing decisional capacity within the context of dementia. Someone may lack decisional capacity due to being intoxicated, impaired by medication, deathly ill, or being overwhelmed by a traumatic event.

Decisional competence is a legal term. Competence is ultimately decided by a judge, who weighs opinions rendered by court-appointed or court-recognized experts.

How is decisional capacity determined?

Partly by a thorough examination. If memory issues are present, the first thing needed is to identify what parts of the mind are working, and which parts are having trouble. Dementia is more than memory loss. In someone with behavioral variant frontotemporal dementia (bvFTD), the main problems usually involve judgment and control. The person with bvFTD can recall a list of words and count backward from 100 by 7. Yet, the person with bvFTD may struggle with mimicking the examiner's hand gestures or drawing a cube. That person may easily fly into road rage and try to run the "offending" driver off the road or hand a complete stranger a check for $50,000. The part of the brain that controls judgment and self-restraint is slipping away. A person with mild bvFTD may have less decisional capacity for a financial problem than a person with mild vascular dementia.

Once the examiner has a general idea as to which parts of the brain (and what cognitive abilities) are strong and which ones are struggling, the examiner can ask some questions. Let's say the person living with dementia wants to help out an adult child who is struggling financially. The person receiving the handout will likely exclaim that "mom knows what she is doing." The other siblings may express concern: "Is mom being taken advantage of?" One way to gain some clarity is to see if mom understands the problem, appreciates the impact of the problem, understands the pros and cons of the issue, and can articulate her decision and why she made it in a way that shows she systematically thought through the issue. If I were asked to weigh in, I'd ask these questions:

1. What is the problem?

In other words, I would want to ask the person living with dementia, what is going on with your adult children? What is the problem? Compare these potential responses.

Response #1: "Fred lost his job and he is unable to pay his bills. I'm going to give him $10k until he is able to find a new job. I don't expect him to pay it back. I paid for the other two daughters' weddings, I never helped him the way I had helped the girls."

Response #2: "Oh, they are always arguing about something. The girls get angry when I help Fred."

If I received response #1, I would likely say that the person living with dementia understands the situation. If I received response #2, I would have concerns about her decisional capacity for lending money.

2. What are some other options?

I would ask if the person living with dementia has some alternative ideas or solutions. What alternatives were offered by the other children?

3. What are the pros and cons of the proposed action? What are potential consequences (intended and unintended) of the proposed action?

Although the adult children may already know the answers to the following questions, it is helpful to hear the responses from the person living with dementia in order to determine their understanding of the decision. And possible outcomes of the decision on his or her life:

- Does $10K represent the person's entire life savings? Will giving that much money away cause hardship to the individual or future caregivers? For someone with seven figures in investments, $10K is a much smaller percentage than $100K in the retirement portfolio.

- Is this an isolated incident, or is Fred expecting ongoing financial support while he searches for a job?
- Is Fred making promises in exchange for the funds? Promises such as, "I'll always be here to care for you, Mom. I won't let them put you in a nursing home." It may be that the other siblings' concerns about financial exploitation and coercion are founded.

It is interesting to hear what the person living with dementia reports as the pros and cons. She may sorrowfully admit that yes, this is an ongoing problem but she feels guilty if her son is homeless. Or, she may assert that Fred isn't asking her for help, she decided to broach the topic and he accepted.

4. What is the final decision and why?

The challenge here is asking the question so that the person living with dementia does not feel attacked or doubted. Those emotions can cause the person with dementia to stop any discussion with the family. One approach is, "I'm curious what you finally decided to do for Fred." After the person living with dementia gives the decision, a follow-up could be, "OK. How did you get to that decision?"

Bottom Line

For financial matters, it is a good idea to put everything in writing, even if the person living with dementia exhibits decisional capacity for that specific issue. Naming a trusted person as power of attorney is also important. Decisional capacity does not mean everyone agrees with the person's final decision; I can have the ability to make a decision, but may still make a poor one because I allowed emotions to affect my decision or failed to heed good advice.

CHAPTER 26

Stopping Medications

When is it OK to stop two common medications, Aricept (Donepezil) and Namenda (Memantine) for people with Alzheimer's dementia?

The short answer is these medications are designed to slow down the nerve damage from AD. Neither medication treats the disease, just the symptoms. These medications are meant to delay the need for 100% care. Once that happens—once the person is now 100% dependent on others for care—the medication(s) have done their job and can be potentially stopped. PLEASE CONSULT WITH YOUR PROVIDER BEFORE STOPPING THE MEDICATIONS YOURSELF!!

Donepezil (Aricept)

Donepezil (Aricept) is a cholinesterase-inhibitor, meaning that it prevents the body from making the enzyme cholinesterase, which breaks down acetylcholine. Acetylcholine is very important for the making and retaining of memories. In a brain without dementia, nerve cells constantly make chemicals like acetylcholine. The cells then secrete enzymes that break down acetylcholine, suck up the raw materials, and then make new acetylcholine. This process results in a "fresh" supply of acetylcholine at all times.

In a brain with dementia, neurons are dying off. As the number of healthy neurons decrease, the level of fresh acetylcholine also drops because the cells still secrete enzymes to break down the acetylcholine but there are fewer healthy cells to replace the acetylcholine. Donepezil manages to keep the level of good acetylcholine higher than the number of healthy cells.

Acetylcholine, however, does degrade over time. At some point, the Donepezil no longer keeps the levels of acetylcholine high enough and the person with dementia shows more memory problems and more loss in abilities to care for him or herself.

Donepezil Usage and Side Effects

Donepezil is approved for mild, moderate, and severe Alzheimer's dementia. The usual dosage is 10 mg daily; however, it can be given as high as 23 mg daily. The issue with the higher dosages is that the side effects are dose-dependent, while efficacy is less so. This is why you will rarely see the 23 mg dosage. Donepezil *can* result in overall improvement of neuropsychiatric behaviors, *but not in persons 85 years of age or older*. Donepezil is not appropriate for persons with frontal-temporal dementia because these individuals have normal levels of acetylcholine; Donepezil can create an acetylcholine-driven delirium.

Common side effects are the usual ones: GI (nausea, vomiting, diarrhea). Other side effects include bradycardia (slow pulse), dizziness, syncope (fainting), tremors (worse in persons with Parkinson Disease), Dementia—rivastigmine, another type of cholinesterase inhibitor, may be a better choice and is FDA-approved for use in people with Parkinson Disease Dementia), and muscle weakness. The side effects are the result of stimulation of cholinergic receptors in muscle, cardiac, and GI tissues.

Sometimes, older adults are taking medications that cancel each other out while increasing side effects: like taking both a pro-cholinergic medication (Donepezil) and an anticholinergic medication (oxybutynin). **It is always a good idea to bring all of the medication bottles to each medical appointment (especially with specialists who tend to get tunnel-vision) and double-check that new medications won't cause new problems.**

When to Stop Donepezil

Donepezil is prescribed to slow down the progression of dementia. Once a person with dementia requires full-time care, Donepezil may no longer be needed. ONE NOTE OF CAUTION: if the individual with dementia is able to walk around independently or can feed him/herself, stopping the

<u>Donepezil may result in the loss of these abilities.</u> Donepezil at the 10 mg daily dose does not need to be tapered; it can be stopped immediately. Some clinicians think that a taper is needed because of the FDA's recommendation that Donepezil be started at 5 mg for 4-6 weeks before increasing to the daily 10 mg dosage. This recommendation was made because participants in the clinical studies who followed the slower route to the 10 mg dosage had much fewer side effects than the participants whose dosages were increased after a week on the medication. If there is concern about a decline in function or an increase in agitation, the Donepezil can be dropped from 10 mg to 5 mg for a week. At the point, the person should be evaluated and if there are no new problems or behaviors, the medication can be stopped. On the other hand, if the decrease in dosage results in an increase in behaviors or a significant decline (for example, the individual was walking independently but the staff notice problems walking after the dosage was reduced), it may be prudent to return to the 10 mg dosage.

Memantine (Namenda)

Memantine (Namenda) is an N-methyl-D-aspartate (NMDA) receptor ANTAGONIST, meaning it blocks this receptor from being stimulated by other neurochemicals. Chronic activation of NMDA receptors over time contributes to shrinkage of the brain matter—a process known as "excitotoxicity." This excitotoxic pathway is also thought to contribute to the changes in cognition and personality often seen in survivors of traumatic brain injury.

Memantine Usage and Side Effects

Memantine is approved for use in **moderate to severe** Alzheimer's dementia only. When the cognitive test scores decline below the 66th percentile (for example, less than 20 for the MMSE), clinicians often introduce Memantine. Published research is difficult to interpret because of the volumes of publications funded by the pharmaceutical industry. However, I located some solid meta-analyses and integrative reviews that suggest that Memantine can help slow down the loss of cognition in persons who have vascular dementia. Memantine does not help with the dementia-related behaviors. Also, monotherapy (Memantine alone) is better than placebo, **but** the findings are mixed when examining the effect of combining Memantine with Donepezil—even though it is done all of the time.

Side effects include constipation, dizziness, headache, hypertension, and somnolence.

Memantine is available in two forms: a short-acting preparation and an extended-release preparation. Memantine 10 mg twice daily provides the same benefits as Memantine 28 mg extended release. The extended-release formulation, however, usually has much higher co-pays and costs more than the 10 mg shorter-acting formulation. Memantine is usually initiated at 5 mg daily for 7 days, then 10 mg daily for 7 days, then 15 mg daily (10 mg in AM, 5 mg in PM), then 10 mg twice daily. The XR formulation is prescribed as 7 mg for a week, 14 mg for a week, 21 mg for a week, then 28 mg daily.

When to stop Memantine

Like the situation with Donepezil, when a person with dementia requires placement and is no longer walking independently or engaging in any self-care activities, Memantine may no longer be needed. ONE NOTE OF CAUTION: if the individual with dementia is able to walk independently or can feed him/herself, stopping the Memantine may result in the loss of these abilities. Memantine should be discontinued in the reverse order of how it was started. If a significant decline in ability is noted, the person should return to the previous dosage level of the medication. For example, if the individual began having trouble walking when the Memantine dosage was dropped from 10 mg daily to 5 mg daily, the dosage should go back to 10 mg daily—not the original 10 mg twice daily!

Families may fail to see progress and may ask about whether their loved one should be taking Donepezil, Memantine, both, or neither. This is a valid question and the IDEAL SITUATION is for the prescribing clinician to have a conversation family members about goals of care and the risk/benefits of continuing or stopping either medications.

CHAPTER 27

Dementia and NO FILTER!

Regardless of the type of dementia, nearly all family caregivers express concerns about their loved one's lack of filter, especially the use of swear words.

Why do People Living With Dementia Suddenly Start Swearing?

People are shocked when someone who never uttered a swear word or acted inappropriately suddenly begins to do one or both as the dementia progresses. Families are horrified and embarrassed. What is going on? What can be done?

I have a colleague who never used profanity in my presence. One day, I asked his opinion about a specific physician that my mother was going to see. "Great surgeon, but a total asshole otherwise." I was caught off guard and blurted, "I didn't think you even knew that word!" People have knowledge of many naughty words but can CHOOSE not to swear or use vulgar language. This choice involves the front and side part of the brain, the frontal and temporal lobes. This choice is influenced by culture, upbringing, cohort (e.g. baby boomers versus millennials), even geography. Here is a fun activity: listen to music from the 1950s to today. Any profanity in 1950s and 1960s music? Nope. How about 1970s? Maybe a "bitch" here or there. 1980s? Getting spicier. 1990s? Some of M&M's songs are nothing but bleeps!!! 2020s? Yeah...you get the picture.

Speaking of choice, I love to watch Gordon Ramsey with the munchkins on Junior Master Chef. He is so well-behaved! Then I watch him with adults and, compared to Chef Ramsey, call me Sister Rita. In my case, I choose to use profanity as a stress reliever, especially when driving. Or to make a humorous point and remove some emotional charge when addressing a deadly serious topic like dementia—which is why this book has a sprinkling of strategic cuss words. At other times, I choose to exert control and use phonetic substitutions like "sugar" or "fudge" for naughty words. My emotions, however, can override my self-control. Literally. A couple of weeks ago, I was riding my horse and we were going over jumps. Jumps are both terrifying and exciting, so I am always super emotionally charged during these lessons. As Zydeco and I thundered toward a vertical line, Zydeco suddenly ducked right and sped past the jump before I had a chance to react! I was simultaneously surprised and angry and called him a "fucker" before I realized what had come out of my mouth. The 2 young riders (age 13) in the lesson thought my faux pas was hilarious; I felt horribly embarrassed. This scenario can also happen with persons living with dementia, especially in people who used swear words infrequently. High emotions, like a strong tornado, can plough through the controls and out pops a foul or vulgar word.

Septic Tank in the Brain

I often tell people that the sides of the brain contain word dictionaries. I also like to think that the same parts of the brain have a "septic tank" of sorts where the naughty words and thoughts are kept. People who maintain verbal and behavioral composure have strong boundaries around their septic tank, so there is no leakage or back flow. The strong boundaries are enforced by the frontal and temporal (side) lobes of the brain.

Enter dementia. As neurons die in the brain, especially those in the frontal lobes and temporal lobes, the walls around the "septic tank" weaken. At first, strong emotions push the nasty words out of the septic tank and they flow from the person's mouth. As the dementia worsens, the walls around the septic tank become so weak and leaky that the vulgar words simply ooze out during simple conversations. This behavior is not a poor reflection on the person with dementia, anymore than a backed-up septic tank means the homeowner is a bad person. Shit literally does happen sometimes.

The use of vulgar or foul language, or acting out in a sexually inappropriate way, is often seen early in people with bvFTD because the front and side parts of the brain (the septic tank walls) are the first to go while other parts of the brain stay intact. For people with other types of dementia, the frontal and temporal lobes shrink later in the disease, so you may see this behavior as the person moves into the moderate to severe stages.

Handling Difficult Situations

What do you do if your loved one is using vulgar or foul language, or acting in a sexually inappropriate way? One approach is to engage in public activities at times when the person is the most rested. Tired neurons "give up" faster than rested neurons. That is why you may notice this behavior when the person living with dementia becomes fatigued, such as in the late afternoon, or even early morning following a sleepless and active night. Other strategies include changing the conversation or introducing an activity ("let's pet the dog"). I'm a big fan of business cards handy that read, "My loved one has a brain disease, thank you for your patience," and handing them out. I also suggest avoiding stressful situations like crowds, which may also "use up" any frontal lobe control and result in the septic tank overflowing.

Bottom Line

The bottom line is that this behavior is caused by the disease and is no reflection on the character of the person living with dementia, or the character of the caregivers. Unfortunately, there are a lot of people who judge. Tell them Rita said to go fuck off.

***

Is your faith community wanting to become more dementia-friendly? I can help! Contact me: rita.jablonski@gmail.com

CHAPTER 28

Hallucination, Illusions, Delusions

Hallucinations refer to sights, sounds, and smells that come from inside the brain. Hallucinations are common with Lewy Body Dementia but can happen with any dementia. The person with dementia is seeing, hearing, or smelling stuff that the rest of us are not experiencing. Illusions refer to misseeing (misperceiving) objects that ARE real. So how do you figure out the difference? And does it matter? Yes! Read on...

Hallucinations, as mentioned above, involve hearing, seeing, or feeling something that is not there. When I worked the emergency department years ago, I cared for an older woman who insisted there was an elf sitting on my right shoulder. She wasn't frightened by it. In fact, she waved and talked to it every time I came over to her. By the end of the shift, I was starting to think that I had an elf sitting on my shoulder!

In people living with dementia, hallucinations may arise from changes in the brain and the brain chemicals. Hallucinations may be scary, like seeing a stranger standing next to the bed. Or they can be comforting, like seeing and hearing young children playing in the living room. Sometimes the hallucinations may be more like vivid memories, such as when a person with dementia sees a long-dead family member from long ago.

Delusions are false beliefs usually arising from fears. Sometimes, delusions occur early in dementia as the person tries to make sense out of a situation. For example, a woman with mild dementia always puts her house keys in the candy dish on the foyer table. Today, she places the keys inside a cabinet and immediately forgets that she did so. Because she ALWAYS places her keys in the candy dish, she has multiple past memories of doing so. In her mind, she put the keys in the candy dish and now the keys are nowhere to be found. When she finally locates the keys in a cabinet, she decides that a family member is moving her keys on purpose. As more familiar items "disappear," she may become very suspicious and have delusions of people stealing from her. Persons with dementia may have delusions of poverty ("I have no money in the bank") and infidelity ("he is seeing another woman"). When I'm helping a caregiver dealing with delusions of poverty or infidelity, I often discover that these issues existed in the patient's past. Perhaps the person with dementia experienced a time of limited resources or was married to a previous spouse who was unfaithful.

Illusions happen when a person with dementia misinterprets actual objects in the room. A throw pillow is a cat. A garden hose is a snake. Poor lighting that creates more shadows can also create illusions. A shadow on the floor may be misinterpreted as a hole.

"Normal" Illusions

Take a look at the picture on the left. Do you see a pretty vase? Or two profiles gazing at each other? Look again, and you will notice you can "flip" between images. Our brains can see, or perceive, multiple aspects of one picture. This is normal, and you can have fun with it. An illusion is some-

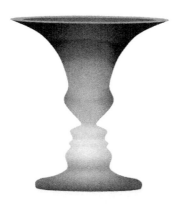

thing that can be misinterpreted by your vision or hearing. Here is another example, something that happens all of the time in the real world. I walk into a darkened room, and before I turn on the light, I become immediately frightened by a scary shape in the corner. As soon as I turn on the light, I see that it is a large plant. Because of the shadows, I mistook the plant for a human figure.

Illusions and Dementia

People living with dementia may experience "breakdowns" in the high-ways that connect different parts of the brain (see Chapter 7). The connections in the brain help us to identify what we see. When I see a furry animal with whiskers, 4 paws, and a tail, my brain tells me that I am seeing a cat. But when the highways slow down or break down completely, I may look at something and my brain connects what I am seeing to something else. For example, I was caring for a relative with dementia who lived with me. She was convinced that the white throw pillows on my black couch were dogs. Sleeping dogs. I suggested that she come over to the couch and see that the objects were pillows. Nope. She was afraid of dogs. So I took the pillows to her. We laughed. She also had some eye problems and wore glasses, so part of the issue may have been distortion due to physical reasons (and smudged glasses).

Illusions or Hallucinations?

One day I received a telephone call from a caregiver who was upset because of her dad's hallucinations. "He keeps seeing men in the house. He won't settle down, he keeps looking for the men and he wants me to call the police." I asked her a couple of questions and found out that the "men" appeared after dark and in specific rooms.

"Do these rooms have windows?" I asked.

"Yes."

"Do the windows have curtains?" I was sure she thought I was goofy, but she was patient with me.

"Yes, but just along the top half. The bottom halves are uncovered. We live in a wooded area with complete privacy, so we don't have to worry about people looking in."

I instructed the daughter to walk through the rooms and see if she could see her reflection in the darkened windows while the rooms were brightly lit.

"YES!" she excitedly answered.

Turns out, dad was NOT hallucinating. He was seeing his distorted image in the uncovered windows, which became funhouse mirrors once it got dark outside. His daughter promptly had shutters installed. Problem solved. Good lighting and removing clutter are two ways to reduce the incidence of visual illusions.

How To Handle Hallucinations

Do the Hallucinations Bother the Person with Dementia?

Towards the end of Mary's time with me, she began to sit in her chair and pick at the air. I watched her one day, and asked what she was doing.

"I'm pulling the yarn down from the ceiling," she calmly replied. She was seeing shiny strands of brightly colored yarn and was delightedly harvesting them. Apparently, she was going to use them in a future arts and crafts project. Her son was freaked out by her hallucinations and demanded I "call someone" to get her medication. I refused. The hallucinations were not bothering her, so they were not bothering me.

Creative Problem-Solving

Another family caregiver shared his story with me. His wife (who had dementia) would stand at the kitchen window every day to look at the birds. This was something she enjoyed. One day, she became upset and told him that a man was sitting in the tree looking in the house. The husband gazed out the window but all he saw was a lone branch jutting off the trunk of the tree. He replied, "Honey, I don't see anything." He suggested that they move away from the window and go do something else in another part of the house. This went on for about a week, with his wife becoming increasingly upset. He simply cut down the tree branch. The hallucinations stopped. Maybe his wife did have visual hallucinations. Maybe his wife was looking at the leaves around the tree branch and was seeing an illusion of a person.

Are Medications Appropriate?

If the hallucinations are scary and upsetting, medications may be warranted. Usually an atypical antipsychotic, and yes, I know these medications get bad reps because they are being used off-label. However, if the medication reduces the scary and upsetting hallucination, and the person with dementia is no longer scared and upset, I think the use of the medication is appropriate. This is a conversation to have with your loved one's dementia care provider.

Delusions

Delusions are difficult to handle. I work with families on a case-by-case basis to come up with a strategy. I have found that keeping the person with dementia on a daily schedule, providing meaningful activities, and utilizing respite care services often "derail" the delusion.

Bottom Line

It's important to figure out if the person living with dementia is hallucinating or perceiving illusions due to lighting and clutter. If the hallucinations are not bothering the person living with dementia, I leave things alone. If the person living with dementia asks me about the hallucinations, I reply that I do not see or hear what they are seeing. If the person living with dementia is upset by the hallucinations, I will add that "this feels very real to you." Delusions are trickier. Some delusions can be understood by recognizing that the person may be moving back in time and re-experiencing troubling memories.

***

I dive super deep into this topic in my dementia behaviors coaching and training programs. You can find out more by going to http://makedementiayourbitch.com or follow me on Facebook→Make Dementia Your B!

CHAPTER 29

Unwelcome Sexual Overtures

Sex and intimacy are topics that are not often encountered in books about dementia, but I wanted to broach it after receiving an email from a reader. Her husband has Alzheimer's dementia and continues to become deeply forgetful, moving backward in time.

In **his** world, in **Dementia Land,** they are young newlyweds, and he wishes to shower his lovely wife with physical affection. He asks her several times a day to join him in the bedroom. At night, he invites physical intimacy. In **her** world, known as **Our Reality**, they are in their late 70s and the physical act of intimacy is something that faded away some time ago. In fact, the physical act of intercourse is painful for her. She loves her husband dearly and does not want to upset or hurt him.

This is new behavior, and she wrote to me because she was very embarrassed and felt alone. With her permission, I am sharing my response because I believe there are others out there who may be experiencing a similar situation. I also encounter this issue regularly in my clinical practice.

New Medication? Recent increase in medication dosage?

Some medications can trigger hyper-sexuality in persons with dementia. These medicines are used with persons who have movement disorders and include what are known as dopamine agonists—such as leva dopa or Sinemet (trade name). Based on what the wife was describing, I do not think medicine is the issue in this particular case. I did, however, encounter a case study in the literature in which a male with dementia was taking cimetidine (Tagamet) and developed hyper-sexual behavior.

What I see in the majority of my male patients is moving backward in time and reliving memories of their youth. The concurrent shrinkage of the brain responsible for impulse control seems to "ramp up" the behavior. The reader described that in her email to me—he thinks he is 18 again, and they are on their honeymoon. He even asks about her wanting to have children! Add to this recipe his lack of short-term memory, and you have kind of a memory-loop. Think of a broken record, where the same piece of music plays over and over again because the needle can't jump out of the groove to the next section of the record.

Knowing the "why" behind the "what" is good—but the next piece, how to handle the behavior, gets a bit tricky. This is a topic that I continue to help spousal caregivers with and I do not have all of the answers. Spouses often find it helpful to enter Dementia Land and respond without arguing: "I love you, too." One caregiver found that giving her husband hugs and kisses was enough to reassure him.

Another one of my spousal caregivers was faced with a husband who would literally ask 10-plus times a day, "Honey, can we go lay down?" This was his euphemism for sex.

She would smile, give him a hug, and say, "OK, after we do [insert chore]."

Here is how their day played out. As they were eating breakfast, he would ask, "Can we go lay down?"

"Sure, right after we wash the breakfast dishes. Can you help me?" He would dry the dishes with her.

Twenty minutes later, he would ask the same question. Her response: "Sure, right after we do this laundry. Can you help me?"

The wife would never say no, she simply redirected him and combined every verbal response with a physical act of love or support: a hug or a squeeze of his hand.

Part of their routine was a nap every afternoon. When they lay down together, he would make romantic overtures. She would tell him that she had her period and could not have intercourse because she felt sore, but she would be happy with kissing and cuddling. This response usually worked, and he often dozed off immediately after laying beside her.

Once he fell asleep, she would get out of bed and let him continue to doze. For some reason, he did not introduce any sexual requests for the rest of the day until after dinner, and she used the same strategies until bedtime.

Adult Children Mistaken for Spouses

Mis-identifying adult children as spouses is not uncommon. Male adult children may be mistaken for their dead fathers by mothers affected by dementia. Female adult children may be mistaken for younger versions of current wives. If a woman or man with dementia acts romantically toward an adult child, this is not incest. It is mis-identification.

Ms. M. was caring for her father with Alzheimer's dementia. Her mother was physically unable to assist with bathing and dressing. Ms. M., in her mid-40s, was horrified when her father tried to passionately kiss her after she had helped him dress. Ms. M. asked me, "Do you think he is some sort of sexual predator and hid it all these years?"

No. I asked Ms. M. to find a picture of her mother in her mid-40s. I asked her, "Is there a resemblance?" Ms. M. was surprised: "We could be sisters! We look so much alike!" I further explained that Ms. M.'s father was moving backward in time. As he lost memories, he probably thought he was in his 40s. In his world, Ms. M. was a small child and his wife was the one helping him dress and bathe. I also asked about the current relationship between Ms. M.'s mother and father. Ms. M. shared that her mother was "in caregiver mode" and all the interactions were clinical, not familial. In other words, Ms. M.'s mother was not acting like a wife—she was not talking with him, reminiscing, joking with him, giving him hugs. She was acting more like a nurse: handing him medications and taking him to medical appointments. This means that Ms. M.'s mother had a "clinical" vibe, not a loving vibe— this was no fault of Ms. M.'s mother; she was unaware that this had even happened. Ms. M.'s father, on the other hand, felt the vibe shift. The change in energy, coupled with her father's memory losses, created a perfect storm where Ms. M. was being mis-identified as her mother.

Ms. M. was greatly relieved by my explanation. I suggested that Ms. M. involve her mother with some of the care, especially intimate care. Ms. M. provided some ideas where she could help her mother balance the caregiver vibe with the wife vibe.

We are all sexual beings and we all want to feel wanted and loved.

Increased sexual behavior may be one way for the person living with dementia to communicate, "PLEASE DON'T LEAVE ME," "AM I STILL LOVABLE?" or "YOU are the ONLY THING that makes sense in my world."

So far, my female caregivers have all developed strategies to manage the behavior in a way that is comfortable for them. We have not used medication to manage the behavior, although the literature does make suggestions for prescribing female hormones to curb aggressive sexual behavior. That is not something we have had to address (yet). I found a case study where the use of citalopram (Celexa, an anti-depressant) curbed this behavior. I do prescribe Citalopram frequently in my practice for underlying depression—I'm not sure if that that drug is helping with the behaviors.

The person who first emailed me responded that my information was helpful. She was happy to know that she was not alone, that others also experienced this situation.

I have to offer a word of caution—what I described occurred with individuals who had been diagnosed with Alzheimer's Dementia. There are hyper-sexual behaviors that can occur with persons diagnosed with bvFTD but that is beyond the scope of this book.

Bottom Line

All behaviors in Dementia Land are meaningful and represent ways that deeply forgetful persons communicate their feelings, needs, and fears. As caregivers, we enter their world and figure out the message.

What about people living with dementia and sexual activity?

This is a tricky area. I know of couples that continue to have intimacy and one has dementia. Unfortunately, I have seen couples where the person living with dementia was expected to participate in sexual activity, and it was clear that they did not want to. Sometimes, people living with dementia who reside in long-term care facilities pair up. These individuals may have living spouses. There are ethical issues and concerns about the ability of the person living with dementia to provide consent. Every situation needs to be considered on a case-by-case basis, which is beyond the scope of this book.

***

I dive super deep into this topic in my dementia behaviors coaching and training programs. You can find out more by going to http://makedementiayourbitch.com or follow me on Facebook→Make Dementia Your B!

CHAPTER 30

Male Caregiver Challenges

Caregivers face many challenges. Hopefully, this book addressed the majority of actual and potential challenges. More importantly, this book provided strategies and approaches for many dementia caregiving challenges. The majority of caregivers are women. In this chapter, I discuss some unique challenges faced by male caregivers.

Men seem to have a more difficult time with the role of caregiver. There are many published studies that examine the differences between men and women who are caregivers. Often, the gender differences are often affected by the relationship between the caregiver and the care recipient. My interactions with male caregivers over the past 10 years have helped me modify my coaching approaches to them.

CAUTION: I do not intend to over-generalize or over-simplify. I understand that people are individuals. However, I've noticed some trends both in my own practice and research, coupled with information from published research studies, that are influencing how I approach caregivers. Hopefully, in an improved manner that better matches their needs.

Mr. Fix-It

Men tend to be problem-solvers, probably from a combination of social, culture, and environmental factors. I'm seeing this with my own son:

Situation: Broken Toilet

Me: "Oh, shit. Something else to handle."

Son: "Yay, trip to Home Depot!!"

Again... just an observation.

The problem-solving approach works with many of life's problems. There is a logic to problem-solving that involves deduction and reasoning. In the case of the troublesome toilet, Mark and I noted that the toilet kept running, which caused us to peek under the tank cover. We saw the broken 'innards' and Mark happily ran to Home Depot and obtained the pertinent parts. Ten minutes later, he replaced the broken components, and everyone was happy.

...And then there is Dementia Land.

There is a logic, all right—but the logic comes from the experiences and memories of the person with dementia. It is a lot like a personal organization system: my spice rack is organized by the ones **I** use most frequently; when Mark is on cooking duty, he fusses because "your organization makes no sense." *NO, SON. IT MAKES PERFECT SENSE TO ME. YOU ARE JUST ANNOYED BECAUSE YOU CAN'T FIND THE CINNAMON.*

Many of my male caregivers, at least in the beginning, **are trying to fix the dementia.** They believe that by quizzing, making the person draw a clock, and employing a range of other activities, they will stop or slow the decline. Some activities have been shown to slow declines in both mental activities and functional abilities (see chapter 12). BUT, they have to be pleasurable and meaningful for the person with dementia or you are going to have a MAJOR behavioral problem. Or several.

Mr. Self-Fix-It

When I work with male caregivers, I emphasize the need for them to use these same problem-solving skills, but on THEMSELVES. The person with dementia cannot function in our world, we are best served entering theirs.

We talk about common triggers of yucky behaviors (refusals, arguing, anger). These triggers are often tone of voice, long/multiple sentences, and other mannerisms that can be seen as bossy. *These triggers are more pronounced when the caregiver is an adult child of the person with dementia.*

- Tone of voice. Make sure you are not using high-pitched baby talk or authoritative (bossy) tones

- Approach. Smile, even if you are not feeling it.

- Short, sweet, concrete. Keep your statements brief and goal-focused. Instead of, "Do you want to get out of bed today?" try "Time to get up." It is much preferable to repeat the same 3-5 words over and over, than to keep restating the same direction multiple ways.

- Give a reason that MAKES SENSE TO THEM. Everyone needs a "why." Think about your own lives. I get out of bed at 4:45 am because I want to accomplish things that make me feel happy and productive. I work late when I'm under a deadline. Those are my "whys". What "whys" would make sense to your family member? Use their past professions or favorite hobbies. Was your mother an attorney? "Mom, time to get up. The trial is today." Was your wife an educator? "Hon, time to get up. The students are waiting." **You are respecting your loved one by bringing a cherished identity back to them.**

"I Didn't Sign Up for This"

Women have historically outlived men, so we as a society are very comfortable with female family caregivers. Most of us women have been socialized to be caregivers in some way, shape, or form. Some women are absolutely NOT cut out to be caregivers in spite of societal and cultural expectations—that is content for another day. Likewise, many men may not have pictured themselves in this role, and most are happily surprised to learn that they are really good at caregiving. But... and I see and hear this a lot...

"This isn't how it was supposed to be."

"I didn't sign up for this."

Many men struggle with the disconnect between the life and situation they expected versus the life and situation they have now. This disconnect is even more pronounced if the male caregiver had physical problems and the spouse was physically helping him before the dementia arrived. Suddenly, the male care recipient becomes the caregiver. These individuals may benefit from more support, especially hands-on support, from friends and family. **This is the time for friends and family members to offer real, concrete help such as dedicated relief care (I'll stay with her so that you can get to your doctor's appointment.)** The caregiver may initially refuse, "Oh, it's OK." Be persistent; ask if the caregiver has alternative ideas or ways that you can help.

The "Default" Caregiver

Sometimes, the male adult child becomes the "default" caregiver because he happens to be single at the time, is the only offspring living in the area, or is the only child, period. If the relationship between adult child and parent was difficult or strained pre-dementia, it can become even more difficult now. Past issues are not going to be resolved now, no matter how hard you try. The person with dementia is very likely to repeat old (learned) patterns of behavior. A good option is to seek counseling for yourself and work things out for your benefit.

A Final Word...

Researchers are VERY interested in finding specific ways to help male caregivers. One obstacle I see time and time again is that male caregivers are difficult to reach. It's a "chicken or the egg" problem. Many support and educational programs are used predominantly by female caregivers or caregivers. In turn, these support and educational programs tend to become more "female-focused", not out of purposeful exclusion but because of the large number of women who use these services. I would love to hear from support groups or services that significantly help male caregivers or caregivers of persons with dementia. I would be happy to post these resources on my blog and podcast!! Email me at rita.jablonski@gmail.com!

CHAPTER 31

Caring for Adult Children With Dementia

"I Thought I Would be the One Needing Care"

I'm seeing this more and more in the clinic; parents caring for adult children with dementia. The person with dementia is about 50 years of age. The diagnosis may be early-onset Alzheimer's dementia or frontotemporal lobar degeneration (frontotemporal dementia or primary progressive aphasia). The person with dementia has no spouse, no siblings (or siblings unable or unwilling to step in), and no children. The caregiver is a parent who may be 75, 80, or 85 years old... and who may have significant health care issues of his or her own.

To be clear, there is such a thing as "childhood dementia." There is something called Niemann-Pick Disease type C, but I'm not writing about this topic. I am focusing on older adult parents caring for the middle-aged adult children. Not only am I seeing this scenario with greater frequency in the clinic, but I've also been receiving emails and blog comments and Facebook questions about resources for these caregivers. And what I am finding is... not much.

Unique Issues and Problems Faced by Parental Caregivers

All caregivers need to have the necessary legal documents, such as powers of attorney, health care proxies, and advance directives. Getting these documents organized for your adult child, however, does feel weird and scary. The parental caregivers may also want to speak to an attorney about whether or not they need to have legal guardianship. In the case of FTD, where the primary behaviors may be poor impulse control around finances, guardianship is invaluable.

Financial Support and Health Insurance

When people develop dementia in mid-life, there will be a need to obtain disability and health insurance. I have an adult child with severe schizophrenia. It took 3 years to obtain disability, which then qualified her for Medicaid (in my state). Parental caregivers may wind up supporting their child with dementia until these benefits can be obtained. I would also recommend that parental caregivers seek additional legal/financial guidance and advice about accessing their child's existing retirement funds (such as pensions and IRAs); many have hardship and terminal disease clauses for the early release of funds without penalties. Assuming that the child has these assets. I also highly recommend that parents consult legal entities such as Alabama Family Trust. Well-meaning parents may make financial decisions that could jeopardize their child's eligibility for disability or Medicaid.

Contingency Care Plan

Every caregiver must have a contingency plan in the event that they die before their care recipients. However, if I am caring for my mom or dad with dementia, the likelihood is that they will go before I do. I don't feel the pressure that a parental caregiver may feel. There is also the issue of the parental caregiver requiring a hospitalization or becoming incapacitated by a fracture or illness. While all caregivers and caregivers have to think about and have a Plan B (or C, D, etc.), this issue is even more pressing for parental caregivers. Parental caregivers may also want to consider increasing their life insurance coverage and setting up clear arrangements for disbursements in their will.

Support Groups That "Get It"

Support groups can be a wonderful thing, but if you are the only parental caregiver, you may feel even more isolated. The parental caregivers feel lost in traditional support groups. Sure, you can pick up some hints about handling refusal behavior. But caregiving is more than figuring out how to handle difficult or bizarre behavior. It feels great when you know others are going through the same thing.

No Resources? Time to Develop Them

The dyads that are missing from all of the web sites and FaceBook pages and other support services are **parental caregivers for adult children with dementia**. I was unable to locate anything on the various associations' web sites specific to parental caregivers.

Are you a parental caregiver for someone with dementia? Please contact me: (makedementiayourb@gmail.com). Do you know someone who is caring for an adult child with dementia? Recommend this book, recommend my blog, or suggest that they listen to my podcast. Let's get a moderated FB group going or ask me questions (rita.jablonski@gmail.com) and I'll look for answers (or discover them on my own). Share your successes so that you can lift other parental caregivers. We can truly make dementia our bitch as we fight for our kids.

CHAPTER 32

Advance Care Planning & Palliative Care

Advance care planning is important for everyone, especially for those living with dementia. Advance care planning is more than end-of-life care decisions. As people travel on their dementia journey, there are multiple crossroads that involve decisions. Should a person with moderate to severe dementia continue to have colonoscopies and mammograms? The answer depends on what you are going to do with the information. If the mammogram shows a mass, or the colonoscopy shows a tumor, are you going to seek aggressive care like chemo and radiation? Are you and your loved one ready to face faster memory losses from chemo and radiation? Same with colonoscopies. The sedation and the reversal agents can make thinking and memories permanently worse.

This is where palliative care comes in. Many people associate palliative care with hospice care. Those are two entirely different practices. It helps to think of palliative care as optimum symptom management when someone has an incurable disease. Dementia is a terminal disease. There are no cures for dementia, at least not yet. If a person with moderate dementia has knee pain and needs a knee replacement, the palliative care approach would be physical therapy, a supportive knee brace, and pain medicine. People who receive knee replacements must participate in painful and difficult physical therapy, otherwise they never gain sufficient knee flexion and extension. People at the moderate stage of dementia can not independently participate in physical therapy. Therefore, palliative care is a better approach.

It is my practice to have some type of advance care planning conversation at each visit. The conversation may start with the caregiver asking me if mom should have a knee replacement or if dad should have back surgery to address pain issues. As we discuss options, I ask the family members to imagine the post-surgery physical therapy or restrictions. The options are different for a person living with dementia who will participate in physical therapy than for someone who cannot. The conversation also includes the effect of operative sedation and post-operative pain medications on memory and cognition.

As the dementia journey progresses, advance care planning does start to address end-of-life care. Some caregivers have had this conversation with their loved one in the past, and they are clear about their decisions. "Antibiotics are OK, IV fluid is OK, but no breathing machines or CPR."

Other caregivers are troubled. Especially if the relationship between the caregiver and the person living with dementia was difficult. One of my neighbors came to me, and he was clearly distressed. His wife of 10 years (they had remarried in their 60s) developed dementia and was convinced he was not her husband. She called him all sorts of names and fought his attempts to help her. He could not afford 24-hour care or nursing home care. He was exhausted and overwhelmed. When she became seriously ill and was hospitalized, he was paralyzed by his feelings. Yes, she was his wife and he loved her. On the other hand, if she were gone, his responsibilities for her would also be finished. He repeatedly said to me, "I don't want the guilt. I don't want to be the one who killed her." He could not bring himself to agree to any "do not resuscitate" orders.

I reframe advance care planning as allowing natural death when there are no more options. Dementia does more than take away memories. Dementia kills people by killing the neurons that control breathing, swallowing, and wakefulness. Once a person with dementia is bedbound, has problems swallowing, and is asleep more than awake, the dying process has started. The body is shutting down. Putting a tube in the person's stomach is not helpful. These tubes do not prolong life and do not prevent pneumonia. Deciding against putting in a feeding tube is NOT euthanasia, as some groups would have you believe. You are allowing natural death at this point.

I think end-of-life conversations are difficult because we live in a "fear of death" culture. Few of us have ever cared for someone who was dying or who died while we sat at the bedside. I think of the stories my grandmothers told me, of caring for relatives who died at home and then having the funeral in the living room. Now, death usually occurs in a hospital and funerals are held in commercial funeral homes. This fear of death can affect decision making, can stop conversations about end-of-life care and preferences.

For clinicians reading this blog, please start having advance care planning conversations before, or at the beginning, of the dementia journey. Have them at intervals. Advance care planning is not a "one and done" conversation. Preferences change as the dementia progresses. For family caregivers, do not be shy about discussing advance care planning. Talk with your loved one to gain a sense of his or her preferences. Keep the conversation going for as long as you can.

More about palliative care

"Your mother-in-law needs to go to the hospital for a blood transfusion." The call came approximately two weeks after my colleague's father-in-law had passed away and five weeks after her mother-in-law had entered a special care assisted living facility (SCALF) with a dual diagnosis of vascular dementia and Alzheimer's disease. Vicki was 8 hours away at a family function and had to make a quick decision. Her mother-in-law, Mrs. W., had been diagnosed 10 years previously with chronic lymphocytic leukemia, a slow-growing form of leukemia and had been without symptoms up until this point. Vicki was in full crisis mode and felt that her only option was to go ahead with the transfusion—whatever it took to save her mother-in-law's life. Vicki was unaware of what prolonging her life meant for her.

No physician, nurse, geriatric social worker, or SCALF director had ever mentioned an advance directive or palliative care in the many conversations Vicki (who is also a gerontologist) had with them about her care. The only exception was a conversation lasting five minutes to add a "do not resuscitate" directive to Mrs. W's chart. No one told Vicki that the option of NOT having a blood transfusion might be in mother-in-law's best interest—especially given the need for hospitalizations and exposure to painful needlesticks. No one told Vicki that being on a myriad of prescriptions to treat all of her "health problems" might not actually be in her mother-in-law's best interest. **No one told Vicki that the goal of preserving life might not be the most humane goal.** No one told her anything. She realized that there were three overarching questions that she should have asked regarding the blood transfusion:

1. "Is it necessary?"

2. "What would it mean for her right now and for the future?" and,

3. "What decision would she want me to make?"

It was not until about six months later that Vicki decided to initiate a conversation with her mother-in-law's geriatrician, who seemed genuinely relieved that someone else had taken the lead.

What Vicki did not know at the time was that her mother-in-law could have benefitted from something called "palliative care." **Palliative care is a philosophy of care. The goal is to treat and remove, or reduce, symptoms that are bothering the person who has dementia.** This makes sense for family caregivers. When a family member is diagnosed with any type of dementia, families are faced with challenges for care and symptom management over the course of the disease process—which can be anywhere from 4-10+ years.

Why are caregivers not given the option to choose palliative care?

Because of widespread misunderstanding of what palliative care is, even among dementia experts and clinicians—all who think "palliative care" means "end-of-life" or "hospice" care. Nothing could be farther from the truth. Palliative care can include "end-of-life" or hospice care, but this narrow and incorrect understanding of palliative care restricts opportunities for important advanced care planning conversations to occur early in the disease process. Another erroneous belief about advanced care planning is that it is a "one and done" conversation; it is crucial that the conversations are open and ongoing. As the person diagnosed with dementia moves from being a little forgetful to deeply forgetful and thus goes deeper into Dementia Land, the pace and content of these conversations may change. In the beginning of the journey through Dementia Land, mammograms and colonoscopies make sense. Tight control of the blood pressure and cholesterol levels help to prevent vascular problems from making the memory and function problems worse. But as the forgetfulness deepens, things like mammograms, colonoscopies, and even trips to the neurologist become illogical in Dementia Land. Palliative care or **"aggressive symptom management for maximum quality of life IN THE NOW"** should guide healthcare conversations and decisions. The family caregiver becomes the person who can best describe what is "maximum quality of life IN THE NOW" for the person who living with dementia. Without these ongoing conversations, misunderstandings can happen—like it did to Vicki—that result in care that may not be reflective of the wishes of caregivers and persons with dementia alike. The results can include a diminished quality of life or unnecessary and unwanted measures to prolong life.

Caregivers will be faced with clinicians wanting to try a medication, change a medication, or run a test or procedure. The clinician does not know your family member like you do; he or she is trying to help, but the help may not result in MAXIMUM QUALITY OF LIFE IN THE NOW.

We recommend that the caregiver use the following approach for these recommendations with these 3 questions:

1. "Is this (medication, test, procedure) really necessary?" The simplicity or complexity of the medication, test, or procedure factors into this question. A simple blood test or urine test would be better tolerated than an 8-hour sleep study.

2. "How will it maintain or improve my loved one's quality of life in the now?" This second question is a little trickier because quality of life is different for everyone. For my family member, quality of life meant going to church regularly and making needlepoint crafts that she gave away as gifts. For Vicki's mother-in-law, quality of life meant gardening, cooking, and being with her grandchildren.

3. "What would my loved one really want?" If the person is not yet deeply forgetful, you can involve him or her in the conversation. If

the person is deeply forgetful, you will need to rely on your knowledge of the person's preferences.

Physicians, nurse practitioners, and physician assistants are often unsure about when or how to initiate a palliative care conversation. I recognizes that I may be perceived as "giving up" on a person who living with dementia when my intent is the exact opposite. This fear of negative reactions from family members often causes clinicians to procrastinate or even ignore the topic until it DOES become an end-of-life issue. Having dementia does not mean "give up on me." It means that medical and healthcare decisions must make sense in Dementia Land.

The following illustrates this approach; I worked as a nurse practitioner in a long-term care facility in the early 2000s and one of my patients was an 83 year old woman who had had dementia for 8 years. Mrs. S. had been prescribed several medications in middle age to prevent urge incontinence, control her cholesterol level, and to prevent fractures due to osteoporosis. When she was first diagnosed with Alzheimer's dementia, she had been started on Donepezil and later, Memantine. When I began seeing her in the nursing home, Mrs. S. was incontinent of urine and was dependent on others for care, including being fed. I sat with Mrs. S.'s family and recommended that all but a pain medication be stopped. The other medications had out-lived their usefulness and were now posing more risk than benefit. I explained that certain medicines in midlife can lower the risks for heart attacks, strokes, cardiovascular disease, and even kidney problems. But, as Mrs. S. grew older and the dementia worsened, it became more likely that Mrs. S. would die from the complications of dementia, not from heart disease or kidney failure. The family agreed. Mrs. S. lived for 2 more years, and her family believed that Mrs. S.'s quality of life was good.

Alzheimer's dementia and the other dementias are terminal illnesses; people can die from their complications. Medications do not stop the neurons from dying off. No procedures reverse dementia. From a palliative care perspective, every decision is made based on how the treatment will maintain, or improve, the person's ability to enjoy the NOW.

I recommend that family caregivers take a look at "The Conversation Project" (http://theconversationproject.org/starter-kit/intro/), especially the one for Alzheimer's dementia and other dementias. The information relates to end-of-life care, which is only one piece of palliative care. However, it is never too early for ALL OF US to discuss what quality of life means to us personally, and how we would want our end-of-life experiences to be like. The materials provide a starting place for the conversation. As we move along our respective journey through Dementia Land, we need to re-evaluate what quality of life means to the deeply forgetful in our care.

CHAPTER 33

Final Thoughts

Thank you so much for purchasing and reading this book!

I care about dementia caregivers and I really hope this book helped you in some way. I do not have all of the answers. I am sure there are dementia behaviors that I have not addressed. In fact, I thought I was finished this book three different times and then suddenly realized I had omitted a topic that I covered in either my blog or my podcast. If you have a behavior or question that you would like to see addressed in future editions of this book, please email me: info@makedementiayourbitch.com.

While I was writing this book, the FDA approved aducanumab (Aduhelm). I did not include any aducanumab information because I was concerned the information may become stale before this book saw the light of day! I look forward to the day where there is a cure for Alzheimer's dementia and the other dementias.

If you want to work with me, I provide one-on-one caregiver dementia coaching. I am also developing some do-it-yourself courses with monthly question and answer calls. I have a weekly podcast, "Make Dementia Your B*tch," which is available on Apple, Google Play, Spotify, iHeart, Stitcher, and several other platforms: https://anchor.fm/rita-a-jablonski. I am happy to help healthcare companies develop dementia training programs for their employees. I enjoy working with law enforcement and first responders, teaching them about dementia and behaviors that they are likely to see. I can be reached at rita.jablonski@gmail.com .

Printed in Great Britain
by Amazon

46016681R00116